The Complete WEIGHT LOSS WORKBOOK

PROVEN TECHNIQUES FOR CONTROLLING WEIGHT-RELATED HEALTH PROBLEMS

JUDITH WYLIE-ROSETT, EdD, RD
CHARLES SWENCIONIS, PhD
ARLENE CABAN, BS
ALLISON J. FRIEDLER, BS
NICOLE SCHAFFER, MA

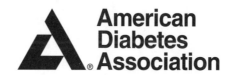
American Diabetes Association

The Complete
WEIGHT
LOSS
WORKBOOK

Book Acquisitions—Susan Reynolds
Production Director—Carolyn R. Segree
Production Coordinator—Peggy M. Rote
Editor—Sherrye Landrum
Designer/Desktop Publishing—Insight Solutions, Inc.
Cover Design—Wickham & Associates, Inc.

Printed in the United States of America

The suggestions and information contained in this publication are generally consistent with the *Clinical Practice Recommendations* and other policies of the American Diabetes Association, but they do not represent the policy or position of the Association or any of its boards or committees. Reasonable steps have been taken to ensure the accuracy of the information presented. However, the American Diabetes Association cannot ensure the safety or efficacy of any product or service described in this publication. Individuals are advised to consult a physician or other appropriate health care professional before undertaking any diet or exercise program or taking any medication referred to in this publication. Professionals must use and apply their own professional judgment, experience, and training and should not rely solely on the information contained in this publication before prescribing any diet, exercise, or medication. The American Diabetes Association—its officers, directors, employees, volunteers, and members—assumes no responsibility or liability for personal or other injury, loss, or damage that may result from the suggestions or information in this publication.

American Diabetes Association
1660 Duke Street
Alexandria, Virginia 22314

Table of Contents

Section Five APPENDICES

Acknowledgements

Project Investigators at the Albert Einstein College of Medicine

Principal Investigator
Judith Wylie-Rosett, EdD, RD
Director, Demonstration and Education Programs, Diabetes Research and
  Training Center

Co-investigators
Charles Swencionis, PhD
Director, Clinical Health Program at Ferkauf Graduate School of Psychology
  of Yeshiva University

Christopher Cimino, MD
Director, Computer Based Education

Sylvia Wassertheil-Smoller, PhD
Division Head, Epidemiology and Biostatistics

Project Director
C. J. Segal Isaacson, EdD, RD

Clinical Project Staff
Arlene Caban, BS, Amanda Cox, BA, Mindy Ginsberg, BA, Maria Kalten, BS,
Kristen Kingsley, MA, Lee-Ann Klein, MS, RD, Ginger Lioi, Alana Riss, BA,
Nicole Schaffer, MA, and Allegra Steinman, BA

Workbook Writers
Arlene Caban, BS, Allison Friedler, BS, CHES, and Nicole Schaffer, MA

Workbook Reviewers
Laura Green, MA, Robert Jeffery, PhD, Elise Sinigra, MS, RD, Madelyn
Wheeler, MS, RD, CDE, Samuel L. Abbate, MD, David B. Kelley, MD,
Connie Crawley, MS, RD, LD, John Devlin, MD, Eva Brzeninski, MS, RD,
and Janine C. Freeman, RD, CDE

Special thanks to Michael Peters, PhD, Yasmin Mossavar-Rahmani, PhD,
Charles Busch, PhD, and Elizabeth Walker, DNS, RN, CDE, for their input.
We thank the participants and staff of Community Health Plan.

Development of the *Workbook* was funded in part by National Institutes of
Health grants No. R01HL39032 and 5P60DK20541.

Preface

This *Workbook* has been used by more than 1500 people to lose weight in National Institutes of Health research studies. Participants have used the workbook to help them learn how to change their lifestyles to be healthier. They learned new ways of eating, how to be more active, and how to deal with stresses that are associated with trying to live healthfully.

In the *Dietary Intervention: Evaluation of Technology* study, older adults used the *Workbook* to learn how to make lifestyle changes to lose weight and be healthier. Study participants lost weight and reduced their fasting blood sugar (glucose) levels. Completing more worksheets in the *Workbook* resulted in losing more weight. The study participants reported being able to continue with their lifestyle changes over a three-year follow-up period and maintained their weight loss and reduction of fasting blood sugar levels.

In the *Trial of Antihypertensive Intervention and Management*, the *Workbook* was used in combination with group weight-reduction classes. The average weight loss was 10 pounds. Interestingly, study participants who lost 10 pounds were more likely to have their blood pressure controlled with a lower dose of medications, and many no longer required any medication to control their blood pressure.

The *Workbook* was revised for the *Models of Demonstration and Evaluation of Weight Loss Study* so it could be used either as a self-help manual or as part of a computer-based, multi-media program guided by a health care professional. The Workbook provided techniques for making lifestyle changes, and the health care professional provided guidance for dealing with more complex health and lifestyle issues. People who worked with a health care professional, such as a registered dietitian (RD), lost more weight in 1 year than those working alone.

The *Workbook* is designed to help you tailor your weight reduction plan to your own lifestyle and health needs and to help you succeed over the long-term. The approach is flexible so you can make changes in your habits that become permanent rather than slipping back into old unhealthy habits. We encourage you to begin now. As our research shows, even a small weight loss and becoming more physically fit can make you feel better because you are healthier.

LIFESTYLE
CHANGE

A roadmap to
reach & maintain
a healthier lifestyle

CHAPTER **ONE**

In this chapter, you learn how to use the workbook

- to tailor a weight-loss plan for yourself
- for a 14-week getting-started program
- to reduce your risk for diabetes

Getting Started

Using This Workbook

The *Complete Weight-Loss Workbook* provides a road map to a healthier lifestyle. This healthier lifestyle includes a plan for lifelong weight control. Your map shows you how to plan meals, increase physical activity, prevent emotions from being roadblocks, and change your behavior.

You can develop a plan to meet your own needs. For example, you can choose an approach to planning what to eat based on counting calories, counting the grams of fat, a meal plan using food exchanges, or a set meal plan. No single approach is right for everyone, and you'll probably use different methods over time. Get help from a registered dietitian (RD) to design a plan to meet your needs. Many people want to be told what to do when they start a weight-reduction program, but they want more food choices after a while. The more you learn about good nutrition and a healthy lifestyle, the more choices you will have. And the more likely you are to succeed.

This workbook helps you develop skills and learn more about the following areas:

Topics	You will learn how to
Section I	
Chapters 1–3	• Use the workbook
Changing Your Lifestyle	• Identify stages you go through in making lifestyle changes
Section II	
Chapters 4–11	• Select and prepare low-calorie and low-fat foods
Food and Meals	• Choose a monitoring method

Topics	You will learn how to
Section III	
Chapters 12–16 Fitness and Health	• Increase physical activity in your lifestyle
Section IV	
Chapters 17–22 Habits and Emotions	• Reduce risks for diseases • Exercise safely • Set realistic goals • Analyze your behavioral patterns • Avoid attitude traps • Develop a support system • Deal with feeling discouraged

Getting Ready for Lifestyle Change

You may have tried to lose weight in the past, or this may be your first attempt to control your weight. Sometimes you may want a rigid plan to follow. Other times you may want more flexibility or control over decision making. No matter what you choose, the process will help you learn more about yourself and increase your ability to succeed over the long run.

Weight control involves more than reducing calories. Your knowledge, approach, and attitudes toward food choices, physical activity, and relationships with others all affect your ability to maintain a desirable weight. The *Complete Weight-Loss Workbook* helps you identify and work on areas that interfere with your goals for losing weight and keeping it off.

Your 14-Week Program

Do not be discouraged if this workbook looks overwhelming—read on! We provide a calendar to follow so that you can read chapters and do worksheets on a weekly basis. You'll see that you don't have to do the chapters in order. You don't have to follow our schedule either, but you may find it makes things easier for you.

The most important part of beginning a weight-loss program is to start keeping a diary. Writing down all the foods or beverages you have daily may not seem important, but your success in keeping a food diary can predict your success in losing weight.

The blank spaces are for you to record the date and to check off what you have completed.

Week 1 _____ *date*

❑ Read chapters 1, 2, and 3 to introduce you to the program and find out whether you are ready.
❑ Complete worksheet 3A: Are You Ready to Lose Weight?
❑ Start keeping a food diary. Look at chapter 6 for help with this process.
❑ See chapter 5 to select a calorie level from the chart on page 26.

Week 2 _____ *date*

❑ Read chapter 5.
❑ Complete worksheet 5A: Your Annual Weight-Loss Record.
❑ Complete worksheet 5B: Patterns of Weight Loss.
❑ Complete worksheet 5C: Measurements.
❑ Remember to keep your food diary. Learning about your eating habits increases your awareness.

Week 3 _____ *date*

❑ Read chapter 6 to help you plan and monitor your meals by either counting calories or budgeting fat.
❑ Read chapter 7.
❑ Complete worksheet 7A: Problem Foods.
❑ Complete worksheet 7B: Using the Exchange System.
❑ Complete worksheets 5A and 5B.
❑ Record what you eat in your food diary.

Week 4 _____ *date*

❑ Read chapters 12, 13, and 14 to help you begin your exercise program.
❑ Complete worksheet 13A: Seeing Your Doctor.
❑ Complete worksheet 14A: Stages of Change.
❑ Complete worksheets 5A and 5B.
❑ Continue keeping a food diary and begin the exercise section of the diary.

Week 5 _____ *date*

❑ Read chapter 4 to learn about the ABCs of eating.
❑ Complete worksheet 4A: What Comes Before Eating—Antecedents.
❑ Complete worksheet 4B: Eating Behaviors.
❑ Complete worksheet 4C: What Happens After Eating—Consequences.
❑ Read chapter 15 to help you develop a plan to become more active.
❑ Complete worksheets 5A and 5B.
❑ Record in your food and exercise diary.

Week 6 _____ date

❏ Read chapters 8 and 11 to help you focus on both eating at home and dining out.
❏ Complete worksheet 8A: Recipe Makeover.
❏ Complete worksheet 11A: Take Charge.
❏ Complete worksheets 5A, 5B, and 5C.
❏ Continue to keep a food and exercise diary.

Week 7 _____ date

❏ Read chapters 9 and 10 to help with reading labels and grocery shopping.
❏ Complete worksheet 9A: The Salami Example.
❏ Complete worksheets 5A and 5B.
❏ Keep a food and exercise diary.

Week 8 _____ date

❏ Read chapter 17 to encourage you to set realistic goals.
❏ Complete worksheet 17A: Your Unreasonable Goals.
❏ Complete worksheet 17B: Overcoming Obstacles.
❏ Complete worksheets 5A and 5B.
❏ Continue to keep a food and exercise diary.

Week 9 _____ date

❏ Read chapter 18 to understand about changing your lifestyle.
❏ Complete worksheet 18A: Previous Attempts to Lose Weight.
❏ Complete worksheet 18B: Analyzing Your Own Behavior Chain.
❏ Complete worksheets 5A and 5B.
❏ Continue to keep a food and exercise diary.

Week 10 _____ date

❏ Read chapter 19 to learn about maintaining weight loss.
❏ Complete worksheet 19A: Problem Areas.
❏ Complete worksheet 19B: Physical Activity.
❏ Complete worksheet 19C: Reviewing the Situation.
❏ Complete worksheet 19D: Preventing a Lapse.
❏ Complete worksheets 5A, 5B, and 5C.
❏ Don't fall behind in keeping a food and exercise diary.

Week 11 _____ date

❏ Read chapter 20 to learn about your attitudes.
❏ Complete worksheet 20A: Core Beliefs.
❏ Complete worksheet 20B: Changing Automatic Thinking.
❏ Review and complete the activity on page 159, Ways to Restructure Your Thinking.
❏ Complete worksheets 5A and 5B.
❏ Keep a food and exercise diary.

Week 12 _____ date

❏ Read chapter 21 to learn how to handle your cravings.
❏ Complete worksheet 21A: Weekly Stress Inventory.
❏ Complete worksheets 5A, 5B, and 5C.
❏ Continue to keep a food and exercise diary.

Week 13 _____ date

❏ Read chapter 16 to learn more about aerobic exercise.
❏ Complete worksheet 16A: Fitness Plan.
❏ Complete worksheets 5A and 5B.
❏ Keep your food and exercise diary.

Week 14 _____ date

❏ Read chapter 22 if you are interested in emotional eating.
❏ Complete worksheet 22A: Am I Ready to Stop Bingeing (if it applies to you).
❏ Complete worksheet 22B: My Goals.
❏ Complete worksheet 22C: Problem Solving.
❏ Complete worksheet 22D: Dealing With Those Who Encourage Me to Eat.
❏ Complete worksheet 22E: How Assertive Am I?
❏ Complete worksheet 22F: Managing Your Time.
❏ Complete worksheets 5A, 5B, and 5C.
❏ Don't forget your food and exercise diary.

Reducing Your Risk for Diabetes

What is Diabetes?

When you have diabetes, your body has difficulty converting food into energy. The human body uses blood glucose for energy. Glucose comes primarily from the carbohydrates that you eat. During digestion, carbohydrates are broken down to glucose. Glucose travels through the bloodstream and is used by cells for energy. Insulin, a hormone created by the pancreas, helps glucose get into the cells. If you have diabetes, your body either makes no insulin or not enough insulin to help glucose get to the cells. As a result, the body does not have enough energy to work well, and glucose levels build up in the blood and urine. High levels of blood glucose over long periods of time can cause damage to many parts of the body. That is why people with diabetes want to get their blood glucose levels into normal ranges as often as possible.

Type 1 diabetes usually affects children and young adults. Overall, only about 5–10% of people have this type of diabetes. People with type 1 have to inject insulin, because their pancreases no longer make any.

Type 2 diabetes is the more common form of diabetes. About 90–95% of people with diabetes have type 2 and most of them are more than 40 years of age. People with type 2 make insulin, but their bodies either can't use it or there is not enough for the body to work properly.

Are You at Risk?

For most people, developing diabetes is a gradual process. The risk of developing diabetes increases with age. As people get older, they become less active and tend to gain weight. After age 60, the average American has a 1 in 3 chance of developing diabetes or having a higher than normal amount of glucose in the bloodstream. This can result in another problem called impaired glucose tolerance (IGT). IGT often leads to diabetes, and both diabetes and IGT can lead to poor circulation and cardiovascular disease.

Research shows that your risk for diabetes is higher if you are over 30 years of age, not physically active, overweight, or have a family member with diabetes. African-Americans, Hispanics, Asians, and American Indians are at higher risk for developing diabetes. Overweight women, women who have had a baby that weighed more than 9 pounds at birth, and women who had gestational diabetes during a pregnancy are at an increased risk for developing diabetes.

If you want to reduce your risk of disease and improve the quality of your life, control your weight and increase your level of physical activity. Whether you are at risk for diabetes or not, learning to eat healthfully, being more active, and targeting the emotions that block your success will benefit the quality of your whole life...so let's get started!

CHAPTER TWO

The Stages of Change

Stages of Change

We go through stages whenever we decide to change our behavior. These stages do not always go in sequence. Sometimes you will feel you are moving backward when a roadblock keeps you from making or keeping up with a desired change. The stages of change are listed here:

- **Stage 1:** Thinking about change
- **Stage 2:** Getting ready and taking action to change
- **Stage 3:** Keeping the change

Stage 1: Thinking About Change

You may have considered losing weight after a visit to your doctor, after some of your favorite clothes did not fit, or after seeing how much better a friend feels by achieving a weight goal. Try to be clear about why *you* want to lose weight. If you can't, you may not be ready to change yet.

Ask yourself, "Is losing weight important enough for me to stay on a weight-control program for more than a few days?" If the answer is yes, you are ready to take the next step. If you answered no, stop and think about more reasons for starting a weight-control program. Have people been commenting on your weight lately? Is a loved one nagging you to lose weight? Do you want to lose weight for a special occasion? Who are you trying to lose weight for—someone else or yourself? To be successful, you have to want to lose weight for yourself, not for someone else. You have to be willing to change. Making the promise to yourself to lose weight shows that you are motivated and committed. The strength of this promise to yourself will help you succeed in losing weight and keeping it off.

Stage 2: Getting Ready and Taking Action to Change

Getting ready is preparation. You can prepare by buying a food scale or making a list of nutritious foods to buy. It may take more time to prepare nutritious meals, so you could gather recipes. Planning is an important part of your program. It requires time and effort. (But what a good investment!) You may prepare by writing down a list of "problem foods." These are foods that lead you away from your weight-loss goals. These foods can be challenges, but don't think of them as bad. You can still enjoy them in moderation. Making a list of problem foods and thinking of ways to monitor how much of them you eat can prepare you for success.

Whatever you identify as the first step to take, prepare, and then do it. Practice the new behavior daily. Make it a part of your everyday life. Taking action to change your eating habits requires a commitment to change. If this seems overwhelming to you right now, don't worry. Change comes in small steps. This workbook is designed to help you through the process.

Stage 3: Keeping the Change

The biggest obstacle most people face as they try to change their lifestyle is continuing the positive changes that they have made.

You don't want to slip back into old habits and ways of behavior. Keeping track and keeping things in perspective can help you. You can use the skills you learn in this workbook to continue the new healthier behaviors until they become your habits.

CHAPTER **THREE**

In this chapter, you think about
- weight loss
- the pros and cons of long-term weight loss

Worksheets to complete
- Are You Ready to Lose Weight?

Are You Ready to Lose Weight?

Thinking About Weight Loss

Losing weight and keeping it off is not easy. It is a slow process that requires many little changes. Becoming aware of why you are overweight and taking steps to break old patterns takes motivation and commitment. If you are willing to make a long-term commitment to lose weight, you will.

Pros and Cons of Weight Loss

First, look at the way you eat. Your style of eating can affect your weight-management program, just as your style of driving can affect the performance of a car. Read Dan and Mary's stories. As you read them, think about who you identify with the most.

Delaying Dan

Dan is overweight. He has gained about 20 pounds in the past 2 years. Dan now feels uncomfortable about his weight. Although he wants to change, Dan does not seem ready to start a program just yet. Take a look at the list Dan created to help him decide if he is ready to make the changes necessary to lose weight.

Dan's List

Pros	Cons
Look more attractive	Give up favorite food
Clothes would fit more comfortably	Begin exercise program
Wife would be pleased	Give up drinking with friends
	Give up snacking in front of the television set
	Constant effort

Dan's list of concerns (cons) outnumber his preferences (pros). He needs to think more about why he wants to lose weight before he attempts to change his habits.

Motivated Mary

Mary has 40 pounds to lose. She feels fed up with the way her extra weight makes her feel. She is tired all the time. Her doctor has told her that the extra weight may be making the arthritis in her knees much worse. She feels ready to get started and to take action.

Mary's List

Pros	Cons
Be able to walk without getting out of breath	Limit sweets
Feel less tired	Begin exercise program
Improve arthritis in knees	Constant effort
Improve back problems	Limit eating with friends
Enjoy buying clothes again	Limit eating out
Feel better about myself	
Decrease risk factors for heart disease and diabetes	

Mary's preferences (pros) outnumbered her concerns (cons) about beginning a weight-management program. Although her current habits will be difficult to change, Mary is motivated to stick with her plan for a longer period. She wants those advantages in her pros list.

Let's review Mary and Dan's stories. When Mary and Dan looked at the reasons they wanted to lose weight, they came to different conclusions. For motivated Mary, the benefits of losing weight clearly outweighed her concerns about changing her current lifestyle. She was able to take control of her eating and achieve her weight goal.

Dan's approach was considerably different. As a result, he continued to gain weight gradually. One of Dan's problems was that he believed that, to lose weight, he would have to give up all his favorite foods. Instead, he just needs to learn to enjoy them in moderation. If Dan would change his beliefs about weight loss, he would be able to achieve his goals, too.

Worksheet 3A: Are You Ready to Lose Weight?

List your preferences (pros) and concerns (cons) about losing weight.

My Personal Pros	My Personal Cons

Now, look over both lists. Which side is longer? If you listed more cons than pros, then you need to reevaluate your commitment to weight loss. Read Mary's story again. Maybe you can gain insight from her.

Think about how you would answer the following questions. This could help motivate you to begin a weight-loss plan.

1. What things do you miss doing that you can no longer do because of your weight or your physical condition?
2. How would it make you feel to be able to do one or more of these activities again?
3. Are there new activities that you would like to try but your weight keeps you from doing?

If you listed more pros than cons, congratulations! You seem motivated enough to move to the next step of successful weight management.

Section Two

FOOD & MEALS

CHAPTER FOUR

In this chapter, you learn about
• your ABCs of eating
Worksheets to complete
• ABCs of Eating: Before, During, and After

The ABCs of Eating

Identifying the ABCs of Eating

One way to think about the stages of change is the ABCs of eating. What do the ABCs of eating stand for?

> **A** = Antecedents (what comes before)
> **B** = Behaviors (what you do)
> **C** = Consequences (what happens after)

Antecedents are triggers that start you eating, for example, a party or restaurant meal, a stressful day at the office, or a family gathering.

Behaviors are your style of eating. You might binge eat when you are under stress. You might starve yourself throughout the day, then make up for your lack of food at night. You might be the type of person who must feel full after every meal, or you might snack all day. Recognizing your style of eating can put you in touch with these habits so that you can control them.

Consequences are the feelings that follow a behavior. How do you feel after you overeat? After stepping on a scale? Are you depressed or upset? Does this lead to more eating?

Leona and Her ABCs

When Leona overeats, she uses the ABCs of eating to evaluate the situation. The triggers (antecedents) for Leona are being upset and skipping meals. Whenever she is upset or angry, she often turns to food for comfort, and she overeats. Whenever Leona skips meals, she often eats too fast while doing other activities. Overeating is her behavior. After overeating, she has to deal with the consequences, which are indigestion and anger with herself because she has lost control.

Try the following exercise to learn more about your ABCs.

Worksheet 4A: What Comes Before Eating—Antecedents

1. When do I generally overeat? ❑ Morning ❑ Afternoon
   ❑ After dinner ❑ Other times? _____

2. Am I with anyone when I overeat? ❑ Yes ❑ No
   If yes, who am I with most often? _____

3. How do I generally feel just before I overeat? ❑ Happy ❑ Upset
   ❑ Stressed ❑ Other feelings? _____

4. Where do I overeat? ❑ At home ❑ Out

5. Were alcoholic beverages around the last time I overate? ❑ Yes ❑ No

6. Does seeing, smelling, hearing, or thinking about a particular food increase my desire to eat it? ❑ Yes ❑ No

7. Do I eat too much after I have gone for a long time without food?
   ❑ Yes ❑ No

8. Am I often involved in other activities when I overeat (watching television, doing work, etc.)? ❑ Yes ❑ No
   If yes, what are the activities I do most often when I overeat? _____
   _____

Answers

1. People tend to overeat at a particular time of day. Using a food diary can help you identify these times.
2. Friends and family are common triggers for overeating. When you are aware of how they influence your eating, you can start changing the situations.
3. If being happy leads to overeating for you, find ways to celebrate without overeating. If being unhappy or stressed is a trigger, try to deal with the feeling directly rather than burying it by eating.
4. Whether you overeat away from home or at home, your diary can help you see the triggers.
5. If you answered yes to this question, realize that alcoholic drinks can be very high in calories. Alcohol can also make you feel hungry.
6. If thinking about a food increases your desire to eat it, read chapter 21 "Coping With Cravings," to learn more about facing this difficult time.
7. If you overeat most often after you have starved yourself all day, you need to eat more often. If you eat balanced meals during the day, you have no reason to overeat. Slow down when you eat. You'll have time to feel full, and you'll stop.
8. Watching television, reading, or working can be a distraction that allows you to overeat. You should concentrate on your meal. Focus on the taste and texture, and enjoy the food!

For information about	See
Question 1	Chapter 6
Question 2	Chapter 11
Question 3	Chapter 20
Question 4	Chapter 11
Question 5	Chapter 11
Question 6	Chapters 18 and 21
Question 7	Chapter 8
Question 8	Chapters 6 and 8

Worksheet 4B: Eating Behaviors

1. Do I eat my food faster than other people around me? ❏ Yes ❏ No

2. Do I usually eat out of containers rather than putting food on a plate? ❏ Yes ❏ No

3. When I overeat, do I enjoy the way the food tastes? ❏ Yes ❏ No
   If no, am I thinking too much about other things? ❏ Yes ❏ No

4. Do I get a lot of pleasure from eating delicious foods? ❏ Yes ❏ No

5. Do I feel out of control when I overeat? ❏ Yes ❏ No

6. Do I eat large quantities of different foods at one time? ❏ Yes ❏ No

Answers

1. Take time to enjoy your food. When you eat quickly, you eat more than your body needs to feel full. If you eat slowly, you don't eat so many calories. Put the fork down between bites. Chew 25 times.
2. If you are not conscious of your overeating until the containers are empty, there are other factors that influence your eating.
3. Putting your meal on a plate is better than eating from a container because it allows you to monitor your serving sizes.
4. If you say no, you are probably too distracted to concentrate on your meals. The 20-minute rule in chapter 8 may work for you.
5 and 6. If you answered yes to these questions, feeling out of control may cause you to eat large quantities of food at one time. Chapter 22 is designed to help you.

For information about	See
Question 1	Chapter 8
Question 2	Chapters 17, 19, and 20
Question 3	Chapters 7, 18, 15, and 17
Question 4	Chapters 8 and 21
Questions 5 and 6	Chapters 20, 21, and 22

Worksheet 4C: What Happens After Eating—Consequences

1. After eating, how do I feel physically? _____

_____

2. After eating, how do I feel emotionally? _____

_____

3. When I overeat, do I feel I have "blown" my diet? _____

_____

4. After I realize I have overeaten, do I tend to continue eating? _____

_____

Your answers to these questions may influence how you want to use this workbook. Section IV in this workbook examines emotions and eating.

Answers

1. If you feel physically sick after you overeat, ask yourself if overeating is worth the discomfort it causes you. Whether you feel physically sick or not, you want to redirect the feelings so you do not feel motivated to eat.

2. If overeating affects you emotionally, it is time to change your lifestyle. Write down exactly the emotions you are feeling before you overeat. _____

   _____

   Now that you have these feelings written down, you can prepare to take action. The following table recommends chapters in this workbook that may help you.

3. You may be too hard on yourself and set yourself up for more overeating. Everyone has a bad day from time to time, and you should not deprive yourself of the foods you enjoy. You do need to monitor how much of them you eat.

4. After you realize you have overeaten, you often eat more. How many times have you said to yourself, "After one more treat, I'll be good." "I've screwed up, I'll begin again on Monday." "A couple of laps around the track will burn off these excess calories." "I am so stuffed, but tomorrow is another day."

   There is nothing wrong with these statements. The problem is that most people do not follow their own advice. They do not stop overeating, they do not try again on Monday, and they often invest more time in eating than they do on the track. When tomorrow comes, they go back to their old patterns. It is time to break the cycle. Read the section on Behavior Patterns in chapter 18 for more information.

For information about	See
Question 1	Chapters 19, 20, and 21
Question 2	Chapters 17, 18, and 22
Question 3	Chapter 19
Question 4	Chapters 15, 19, and 20

CHAPTER FIVE

Rate of Weight Loss

Dropping 10 pounds immediately when you are trying to lose weight would be wonderful, but unfortunately, that does not usually happen. Getting rid of excess fat slowly is the healthiest way to lose weight and the best way to keep it off.

Best Rate of Weight Loss

How fast should you lose weight? Experts recommend losing no more than 1 or 2 pounds each week.

This slow weight loss ensures that you are losing mostly fat and preserving muscle. Muscle tissue burns more calories than fatty tissue. Therefore, the more muscle you have, the more you can eat without gaining weight.

You can plot your weight and measure your progress over the year by using the chart on page 30.

Suggested Calorie Goals for Weight Loss

Your current weight (lb)	To lose 1 lb/week	To lose 2 lb/week
Less than 150	1200 calories* (25–30 g fat/day)	Not advised
150–200	1400–1600 calories (35–40 g fat/day)	1200 calories (25–30 g fat/day)
More than 200	1800–2000 calories (40–45 g fat/day)	1300–1500 calories (30–35 g fat/day)

*If you don't lose weight at this level, it is better to increase your physical activity than to drop too low in calories.

Quitter Quentin—What is Water Weight?

The first week that Quitter Quentin went on a diet, he lost 5 pounds. He was thrilled. When he gained 1 pound back the following week, he became discouraged and stopped his diet. Has this ever happened to you?

What Quentin didn't understand was that, during the first week of his diet, about half of the weight he lost was water weight. The fact that he maintained a weight loss of 4 pounds in the second week of his diet means that he probably "burned" off 4 pounds of fat. He was succeeding!

One reason most people lose water weight in the first days of a diet is because they are using up the body's stored sugar before they burn fat. Stored sugar, called glycogen, holds about four times its weight in water. Another factor that can affect how much water weight people have is the salt in their diet. A high-sodium diet can lead to water retention and the common bloated feeling. Eat less sodium and you'll lose water weight.

How Rapid Weight Loss Affects You

Experts recommend that people lose weight slowly. Why? Because rapid weight loss is dangerous. It can cause you to lose muscle as well as fat. This could include muscle that is vital to life, such as heart muscle. If you put weight back on, it is more likely to be fat. This can leave you with a higher percentage of body fat than when you started.

Many people try to lose weight quickly with very low calorie diets. These diets cause the "yo-yo" syndrome of dieting. Read Yolanda and Leonard's stories.

Yo-Yo Yolanda—What is the Yo-Yo Syndrome?

Yolanda is a person caught in the yo-yo syndrome. Her weight had gone up to 180 pounds. She had been eating a little more than 2000 calories a day to maintain her weight at this level. Yolanda went on a very low calorie diet for 8 weeks, eating only 500 calories a day. She lost 40 pounds, much of it muscle, not fat. When she went off the diet, she rapidly regained the weight. Why?

1. Her metabolic rate had slowed down drastically because the calorie level was too low. Her body made adjustments to keep her alive through what it thought was a famine. After her starvation diet, the calories Yolanda needed to maintain her weight had dropped to 600 per day. When she went back to eating regularly, she rapidly regained all the weight she had lost. In fact, she gained an additional 10 pounds before her weight stabilized at 190 pounds.

2. Because Yolanda did not learn any skills to change her eating habits while on the starvation diet, she went back to eating the way she did before.

3. Yolanda lost muscle mass because the calorie level was too low, and she did not exercise. This will make it harder for her to lose weight in the future. *The less muscle she has, the slower her metabolic rate.*

Level-Headed Leonard—Can You Stop the Yo-Yo Syndrome?

Leonard used to be a yo-yo dieter, until he decided that a healthier lifestyle was a better way to manage his weight. Leonard was a yo-yo dieter because

- he used to set calorie goals that were unrealistically low
- he never built exercise into his lifestyle
- he ate very fast

Leonard broke out of this cycle by taking action.

1. He decided that keeping the weight off was important to his health, not just his appearance.

2. He replaced high-fat foods with lower-fat foods.

3. He started parking his car 15 minutes away from his office, which allowed him to build 30 minutes of brisk walking into his busy schedule. Building exercise into his daily routine has been an important factor in Leonard's ability to stay at his goal weight for almost 2 years.

4. He slowed down his rate of eating. Eating more slowly allowed Leonard to enjoy his food and to feel more satisfied with smaller portions.

5. Once a month he weighed and met with his registered dietitian (RD). When he gained 3 pounds, he weighed in weekly and cut back his calorie intake. Because Leonard never allowed his weight gains to become overwhelming, it was much easier for him to maintain his 20-pound weight loss for almost 2 years.

How to Avoid Yo-Yo Dieting

Here are some effective ways to avoid the yo-yo syndrome.

- Lose weight gradually to preserve muscle mass.
- Keep your calorie average above 1000 calories per day.
- Increase physical activity (aerobic and strength training).
- Create a realistic plan you can live with.

Meal plans that are extremely low in fat and calories are not good for your body and are almost impossible to stay on for the rest of your life. Let your progress be gradual. The more gradual your changes are, the longer the results will last.

Obstacles to Weight-Loss Success

You may need to reset your weight-loss goals if you find you are not reaching them at a reasonable pace. An unrealistic plan or an unwillingness to stay with the plan are roadblocks to success.

---

1. Do you say you eat fewer calories than you really do? ❏ Yes ❏ No
2. Are you not exercising regularly? ❏ Yes ❏ No
3. Are particular stressful events or boredom preventing you from following a meal plan? ❏ Yes ❏ No
4. Are you snacking on high-fat foods? ❏ Yes ❏ No

If you answered yes to two or more of the questions, you may find it difficult to maintain the changes in your plan. Sections I and IV focus on how to make lifestyle changes.

Patterns of Weight Loss

It is a good idea to keep a weekly graph of changes in your weight. The amount of weight most people lose each week will vary. The graph can be encouraging because it will show an overall downward trend. It is important to remember that your weight may fluctuate because of changes in fluid balance. If your goal is an average weight loss of 2 pounds per week, you may not lose 2 pounds every week. Instead, you may lose 4 pounds the first week, and gain 1 pound the second week.

Worksheet 5A: Your Annual Weight-Loss Record

Here is another method for keeping track of your weight-loss progress. Each week, when you weigh yourself, record the date and your new weight. This way, you can watch the numbers go down!

Week	Date	Weight	Week	Date	Weight
1.			27.		
2.			28.		
3.			29.		
4.			30.		
5.			31.		
6.			32.		
7.			33.		
8.			34.		
9.			35.		
10.			36.		
11.			37.		
12.			38.		
13.			39.		
14.			40.		
15.			41.		
16.			42.		
17.			43.		
18.			44.		
19.			45.		
20.			46.		
21.			47.		
22.			48.		
23.			49.		
24.			50.		
25.			51.		
26.			52.		

Keeping a graph of weight from week to week is encouraging when you see an overall downward trend. Continue to graph your weight each week until you achieve your goal.

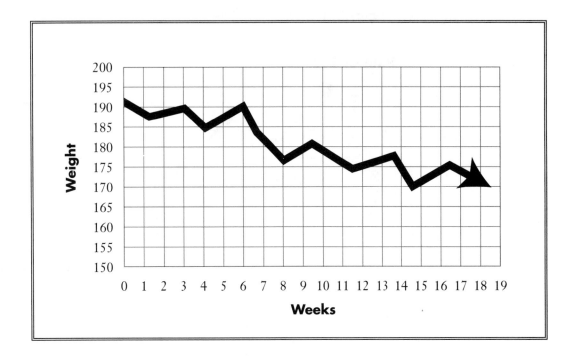

Here's one way to document your weight loss.

1. Put a dot at your current weight.
2. Each week, when you weigh yourself, put a dot to show how many pounds you have lost. If you lost 1 pound, the line between the dots should move downward. If you gained a pound, the line should go up.

Ronald Documents His Weight Loss

Beginning weight ____180____

Pounds Lost

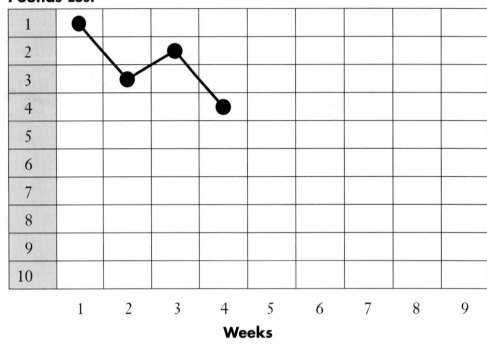

Weeks

In this example, Ronald began at 180 pounds.

1. After the first week of monitoring his meals, he lost 1 pound.

2. After the second week, he lost 2 more pounds (noted on the graph). As you can see from the column on the left, by the second week, he had lost a total of 3 pounds.

3. After the third week, Ronald gained 1 pound. Now the total of pounds lost has changed. It is now 2 pounds.

4. Not discouraged, by the fourth week, Ronald was back on track. He lost a total of 4 pounds in four weeks, even though he had a setback in week 3.

Worksheet 5B: Patterns of Weight Loss

Record your current weight on the weight-loss record below. Weigh yourself on the same day of the week and at the same time so that your measurement is accurate. If you are having difficulty, review Ronald's story.

Beginning weight _____

Pounds Lost

	1	2	3	4	5	6	7	8	9
1									
2									
3									
4									
5									
6									
7									
8									
9									
10									
11									
12									
13									
14									
15									
16									
17									
18									
19									
20									

Weeks

You may photocopy this page for additional weeks. If you want a more accurate display, use graph paper.

Check Your Measurements

It is important to check your measurements once a month. You should measure your chest, upper arms, waist, hips, thighs, calves, and ankles. The scale can't show you the inches that you have lost. When you exercise, you replace fat with muscle and lose inches.

Muscle is heavier than fat. If you see the changes in your measurements, you are less likely to be discouraged if your weight loss is not as rapid as you would like it to be.

For example, Esther only lost 5 pounds in 1 month, but she lost 3½ inches. Two inches were from her upper arms and calves. She would not have recognized her accomplishment if she had not been keeping records of her measurements.

How to Take Your Body Measurements

As a rule, whenever you take your measurements, keep your posture straight, and measure at the widest point. Never wear belts, girdles, or other items that will keep you from getting an accurate measurement.

1. Take your chest, thigh, upper arm, calf, waist, and buttocks measurements in one session.
2. Be sure to measure at the same location each time.
3. Make all measurements while unclothed or in minimal clothing.
4. Always take your measurements while standing. Do not slouch or hold your breath.
5. To measure, start at the 1-inch end of the measuring tape and wrap it around the area you are measuring.
6. Pull the measuring tape snug as you measure but not so tight that you indent the skin.
7. Make sure the tape measure is horizontal all the way around the area you are measuring.
8. Make two measurements of each body part to the nearest ¼ inch. If your measurements are accurate, the two measurements will be the same. If they do not agree, make a third measurement, and record the average on the Measurement worksheet (page 36).

Where to Measure

- **Chest**—at the fullest part after you have exhaled
- **Upper arms**—halfway between the shoulder and elbow
- **Waist**—directly above the navel
- **Thighs**—the fullest part where your leg meets your body
- **Buttocks**—at the fullest part, while you are standing straight
- **Calf**—the fullest part, midway between your ankle and knee

Accuracy, consistency, and honesty are very important if you really want to know how you're doing.

Worksheet 5C: Measurements

Record your measurements once a month on the charts provided.

First month   Date: __ /__ /__
Chest _____   Buttocks _____   Upper arm _____
Thigh _____   Waist _____   Calf _____

Second month   Date: __ /__ /__
Chest _____   Buttocks _____   Upper arm _____
Thigh _____   Waist _____   Calf _____

Third month   Date: __ /__ /__
Chest _____   Buttocks _____   Upper arm _____
Thigh _____   Waist _____   Calf _____

Fourth month   Date: __ /__ /__
Chest _____   Buttocks _____   Upper arm _____
Thigh _____   Waist _____   Calf _____

Fifth month   Date: __ /__ /__
Chest _____   Buttocks _____   Upper arm _____
Thigh _____   Waist _____   Calf _____

Sixth month   Date: __ /__ /__
Chest _____   Buttocks _____   Upper arm _____
Thigh _____   Waist _____   Calf _____

Seventh month   Date: __ /__ /__
Chest _____   Buttocks _____   Upper arm _____
Thigh _____   Waist _____   Calf _____

Eighth month   Date: __ /__ /__
Chest _____   Buttocks _____   Upper arm _____
Thigh _____   Waist _____   Calf _____

Ninth month   Date: __ /__ /__
Chest _____   Buttocks _____   Upper arm _____
Thigh _____   Waist _____   Calf _____

Tenth month   Date: __ /__ /__
Chest _____   Buttocks _____   Upper arm _____
Thigh _____   Waist _____   Calf _____

CHAPTER **SIX**

In this chapter, you learn
- the benefits of keeping a food diary
- how to keep a food diary
- how to plan your meals by counting calories, counting fat, or using a meal plan
- how keeping track reduces risks related to diabetes

Keeping Track of the Foods You Eat

This chapter explores the importance of planning and monitoring the foods you eat.

Benefits of Keeping a Food Diary

Awareness is the key step in changing your behavior. You may think that you know a great deal about your eating habits. You will be surprised at how much you learn from keeping records of what you eat. This activity motivates you and prepares you to change. The best way to keep track of what you eat is by using a *food diary.*

The food diary is the most important tool for changing the way you eat. At first, it may seem to take too much time. But you will soon realize how helpful it is to know exactly the amount and the types of foods you are eating.

Recording what you eat and counting the calories, fat grams, or food groups are the first steps in taking control. Change can begin once you decide to become more aware of your eating patterns. After you make changes in your eating patterns, you will use the food diary less or not at all.

The reasons for keeping the food diary are to

- determine how many calories, fat grams, or servings you are eating
- help you find the most painless way to begin cutting back on calories, fat grams, or servings
- help you become an expert at counting calories, counting fat, or following a meal plan

How to Keep a Food Diary

In your food diary, you need to write down

- the date
- the time you ate
- the meal or snack you had
- how much you ate
- your mood when you ate
- how hungry you felt before you ate
- the number of calories, fat grams, or servings of each food

Under the heading "Calories/Fat," you can keep track of calories or grams of fat. If you have a meal plan, use the form that allows you to check off how many servings you ate. Use the "total" boxes at the bottom of your food diary to record the number of calories, fat grams, or food servings for all the meals eaten in that day.

As you keep records, it is important to do two things:

1. *Measure how much you eat whenever possible.* Use measuring cups and spoons, or calculate the number of servings from the package so that you have an accurate record of what you are eating. Eyeballing a serving size does not work until you have measured the correct sizes for several weeks and are used to seeing and eating them.
2. *Write down everything you eat immediately after you eat it.* You need to carry your food diary with you throughout the day to keep track of everything you eat or drink.

Methods for Planning Your Meals

There are three different monitoring methods you can use in this program—counting calories, counting fat, or meal planning. Read through the preferences (pros) and concerns (cons) associated with each method before you decide which is best for you.

Counting Calories

Some people like the idea of reading labels, using a calorie counter or calculator to keep track of calories, and making lists to stay organized. Other people dread the idea of using a calculator or worry about using math skills to calculate calories. Read the following statements, then check off those that apply to you.

Pros

❏ I want to choose what I am going to eat.
❏ I am interested in learning more about the amount of calories in the foods that I eat.
❏ I am interested in creating my own plan so I can estimate calories.
❏ I want to eat my favorite foods as long as they fit into my daily plan.
❏ I would like to improve my ability to plan healthy meals.

Cons

❏ I have trouble calculating calories, so I may find this approach frustrating.
❏ I may have difficulty making food choices because food labels confuse me.
❏ Looking up foods and recording what I eat each day seems too time consuming to me.
❏ My meals may not be balanced nutritionally. I could eat a lot of fat and stay within my calorie goal, but then I wouldn't be eating enough vitamins, minerals, and fiber.

Review your list of pros and cons. If you checked off more preferences than concerns, then you may enjoy this way to manage your weight. If you checked off more concerns than preferences, then read about other ways to monitor your food intake.

Counting Fat

Some people prefer to count the amount of fat grams they eat, because it is easier than counting calories. People who are always on the go and those who do not have time to keep track of calories by using a calculator often focus on fat. They try to eat foods that have little or no fat (less than 30% calories from fat on the food label). Other people manage their food intake by keeping a closer watch and totaling the number of fat grams that they eat daily. Check off the statements that fit you.

Pros

❏ I enjoy making my own food choices.

❏ I want to create a daily plan that gives me an allotment of fat grams each day.

❏ Fat grams are simpler to compute than calories.

❏ I would feel less restricted if I focused on cutting back fat instead of calories.

❏ It is easier for me to shop because most of my favorite foods have lower-fat versions.

Cons

❏ I may not lose weight as fast as other people who use a meal plan or count calories because I may eat more calories than I am aware of.

❏ There are many new low-fat products on the market that are relatively high in calories.

❏ I do not like the taste of many low-fat and nonfat foods.

❏ Food labels are confusing to read.

❏ My meal plan may not be nutritionally balanced.

Review the list of pros and cons. If you checked off more pros than cons, then fat counting may work well for you. If you checked off more concerns than preferences, then review the other methods, taking some time to evaluate each approach. Choose the method you would be most comfortable with.

Meal Planning

Many people think that using a meal plan is the easiest way to lose weight. If you do not like to make a lot of decisions about the foods you eat, you may like the idea of using a meal plan to lose weight. Many people start off with a fixed meal plan because it requires the least amount of thinking and planning. Other people prefer more flexibility and control over what they eat. They may feel restricted by a fixed meal plan when they eat out or visit with friends and family.

A meal plan organizes foods into six food groups. All the foods in each group have similar numbers of calories and amounts of fat, carbohydrate, and protein.

You can trade one food for another in the same group or exchange them because they are nutritionally similar. To make using the system easier, each group lists a serving size.

Does this sound like the type of monitoring method that you would like to use? Look at the list of pros and cons about using the meal plan. By evaluating your answers, you can decide if a meal plan might work for you.

Pros

❏ I would rather make very few food decisions.
❏ I would like help to resist temptation from foods that are not a part of my meal plan.
❏ I like the idea of monitoring my food intake by marking a tally for each item that I eat from my meal plan.
❏ I like that the meal plan offers a well-balanced diet.
❏ I like that the meal plan ensures that I eat a variety of foods.

Cons

❏ I may feel restricted by fewer food choices.
❏ It may be difficult to follow the meal plan on weekends or special occasions.
❏ I may learn less about how to plan healthy meals.
❏ I may not like the foods on the meal plan.
❏ I may become tired of the foods on the meal plan.

Review your list of pros and cons. If you checked off more pros than cons, then the meal plan approach may work very well for you. If you checked off more cons than pros, review the other two methods of monitoring to identify a better one for you.

You need a monitoring method that helps you keep track of your new style of eating. We have discussed several of your options. You can

- structure your own plan through calorie counting
- structure a plan by counting the number of fat grams in foods
- use a fixed meal plan where you only need to keep track of how many servings you ate from each food group

I have chosen the following monitoring method:

❏ calorie counting
❏ fat counting
❏ meal planning

Now that you have chosen an approach to losing and managing weight, you are ready to develop the skills for weight-loss success. Remember, you can change your monitoring method whenever you want to or if your lifestyle changes.

How Keeping Track Reduces Risks Related to Diabetes

Food plays an important role in managing diabetes. Foods such as fruits, vegetables, milk, breads, grains, and cereals contain carbohydrates that are used by the body to make glucose. They are also part of a healthy diet. If you have diabetes or are at risk for it, improving your eating habits can help you feel better every day and reduce other health risks.

> Avoiding certain foods and sweets will keep you from having problems with diabetes. ❏ True ❏ False

If you answered "True," you need to learn more about how your eating habits affect your blood sugar levels. You can eat sugar as part of a balanced meal plan. The American Diabetes Association 1994 nutrition recommendations stress that there is not a "diabetic diet." What to eat depends on your likes and dislikes, age, sex, physical activity, nutritional needs, and health goals. A registered dietitian (RD) can help you with any questions and tell you how different foods affect your blood sugar levels and your health.

Basically you want to keep your blood sugar levels as close to normal as possible. You do that by tracking what you eat (which raises blood sugar) and adjusting your physical activity and medication, if you take it (which lower your blood sugar).

People with close to normal blood sugar levels have significantly lower risk of complications such as vision or circulation problems. Even after diabetic complications appear, reaching normal blood sugar levels can stop or sometimes improve these conditions. Keeping track of food, activity, and emotions is definitely worth the time it takes.

Blood Sugar Levels

People with diabetes may have highs and lows in their blood sugar levels if they are taking insulin or certain types of oral medications. Lower than normal blood sugar levels, or **hypoglycemia,** is often caused by skipping meals, eating too little, sickness, or increased physical activity.

Higher than normal blood sugar levels, or **hyperglycemia,** is often the result of eating too much, failing to follow a meal plan, sickness, infections, decreased activity, forgetting to take your medication, or taking medications such as cortisone or prednizone.

If you are at risk for developing diabetes, visit your doctor regularly to detect problems early. Many times diabetes is first diagnosed by the appearance of complications that have taken several years to develop. Knowing what factors influence diabetes can help you be more in control of your life.

A Balanced Plan

In this chapter, you chose a self monitoring method to keep track of the fat and calories you eat. Whatever plan you use, make sure it is nutritionally balanced. An RD can help you with this. In chapter 7, you learn more about using the food pyramid for more variety and balance in your meal plan. Appendix B has some sample meal plans and menus to help you, too.

CHAPTER **SEVEN**

How to Plan and Monitor Meals

In chapter 6, you chose a monitoring method after reviewing a list of the pros and cons for each method. Now you can get started on the details.

Complete the section that reflects the choice you made in chapter 6.

Calorie Counting

This section is designed to help you individualize your calorie goal. If you are satisfied with the calorie range in chapter 5 (page 26), then you can go directly to the Problem Foods worksheet (page 49), in this chapter.

To put it simply, you need to decrease the calories you eat by 3500 calories to lose 1 pound. Of course, you can't do this all in 1 day. You can cut your calorie intake by 500 calories each day for 7 days (500 calories x 7 days = 3500).

You can calculate the number of calories you need to eat each day to lose 1 or 2 pounds per week, or you can use the chart on page 26.

Individualized Calorie Goal

You can determine your calorie goal. Your weight depends on how much energy (calories) you take in and how much energy you spend in activity. If we take in more energy (calories) than we burn up by activity, we store the extra calories as fat. To lose weight, you must take in fewer calories or burn up more calories in activity. You learn more about increasing your activity level later in this workbook.

Current Calorie Level

To begin eating fewer calories, you must first know how many calories you need to maintain your current weight. *Maintain* means you don't lose and you don't gain weight. To estimate how many calories you need daily, multiply your current weight by 11. Read the following story to see how this works.

Jason's Calorie Goal

Jason weighs 190 pounds. To determine the number of calories he needs to maintain his weight, Jason multiplies his weight by 11

$$190 \times 11 = 2090$$

Jason requires approximately 2090 calories a day to maintain his current weight.

To lose weight, he needs to eat fewer than 2090 calories.

For Jason to lose 1 pound per week:

$$\text{current calories} = \begin{array}{r} 2090 \\ -\ 500 \\ \hline 1590 \text{ calories per day} \end{array}$$

For Jason to lose 2 pounds per week:

$$\text{current calories} = \begin{array}{r} 2090 \\ -\ 1000 \\ \hline 1090 \text{ calories per day} \end{array}$$

Jason does not want to fall below 1200 calories per day, so he chooses to increase his exercise time to burn off those excess calories.

To determine the calories you need to maintain your weight

Your weight _____ x 11 = _____ current calories

To lose 1 pound per week:
current calories = _____ − 500 = _____ calories per day.

To lose 2 pounds per week:
current calories = _____ − 1000 = _____ calories per day.

Now that you have calculated how many calories to eat each day to lose 1 or 2 pounds per week, which goal is realistic for you? Generally, it is recommended that you lose 1 pound per week. Weight loss should be gradual.

Your Calorie Goal

I think it is realistic for me to lose _____ pound(s) per week, so my daily calorie goal is _____.

Calorie Counting

Calorie counting involves keeping a food diary and looking up the number of calories in foods. You need to write down everything you eat as you eat it. If you wait until later or the end of the day, you may forget what you ate. For example, it's easy to forget that you tasted chocolate at the office or the chips you ate as you ran from one place to another. That's why it's better to keep a running total of your calorie intake. This may be difficult at first but will soon become a part of your daily routine. The running total will tell you how many calories you have left to eat each day.

For calorie counting to be useful, it must be accurate. Calorie information is available on food labels and in calorie books. To determine how many calories you have, you must monitor the amount of food you have eaten.

For example, an extra 2 ounces of meat can add up to 200 calories. Because cuts of meat vary so much in shape and thickness, it is almost impossible to guess how many ounces of meat you have in a serving. You must weigh it. When using the calorie information on food labels, be sure to check the serving size carefully. Manufacturers sometimes list unrealistically small serving sizes, so the calories per serving seem to be less than they really are. Your normal-size serving may have more calories.

Fat Counting

The main source of hidden calories in our diet is fat. Gram for gram, fat has more than twice the calories of protein or carbohydrates.

---

1 gram of fat = 9 calories
1 gram of protein = 4 calories
1 gram of carbohydrate = 4 calories

For example, a 3-oz baked potato with its skin has 0 grams of fat. The margarine or butter that we add to the potato has about 100 calories and 12 grams of fat per tablespoon. The butter has 12 times more fat than the entire potato.

Fat counting involves keeping a food diary and looking up the amount of fat in foods. Fat is the most concentrated source of calories (9 calories per gram). When you cut back on fat, you are cutting back on your calories as well. Your fat budget is figured from your calorie goal for weekly weight loss.

The American Cancer Society, the American Heart Association, the National Institutes of Health, and many other organizations recommend that less than 30% of total calories come from fat. Limiting your fat to 25% of your calories may make losing weight easier. What does this mean for you?

If you are following a

- 1200-calorie plan, limit your fat intake to 33 grams a day
  1200 (total calories) x 0.25 (% from fat) = 300 (calories from fat)
  300 (calories from fat)/9(calories per g fat) = 33 g fat

- 1500-calorie plan, limit your fat intake to 42 grams a day
  1500 (total calories) x 0.25 (% from fat) = 375 (calories from fat)
  375 (calories from fat)/9(calories per g fat) = 42 g fat

- 1800-calorie plan, limit your fat intake to 50 grams a day
  1800 (total calories) x 0.25 (% from fat) = 450 (calories from fat)
  450 (calories from fat)/9(calories per g fat) = 50 g fat

My fat budget has _____ grams of fat.

Many foods are naturally low in fat, such as fruits, vegetables, many breads, pasta, and rice. However, you need to be careful of salad dressings, sauces, and the hidden fats in prepared pasta and rice products. Crackers and muffins are often high in fat, too.

Your food diary helps you keep track of how many grams of fat you eat each day. You can look up the number of grams of fat in foods on food labels and in calorie books. Before you write the number of grams of fat, you must compare your serving to the serving size on the food label. For example, if you ate 2 teaspoons of margarine on your toast but the label indicated that a serving was 1 teaspoon, then you must double the amount of fat grams on the label when you record it in your diary.

Cutting Down Fat

Some fats can be trimmed off the food we eat, like the fat on a steak. Other fats are hidden in foods, like the fat in cakes, cookies, potato chips, nuts, and cheese. (Check the label on **low-fat** versions of these foods. They may be high in **calories.**) Limiting your fat intake has other advantages besides making weight loss easier. A low-fat diet may help lower your risk of heart disease, colon cancer, and breast cancer.

Meal Planning

Meal planning helps you get all of the nutrients you need each day. You can choose a calorie level for your meal plan using the chart on page 46.

The Exchange System

All the menus in this program were developed using the exchange system. The exchange system categorizes food into three main groups—carbohydrates, meat and meat substitutes, and fat. Starches, vegetables, fruits, milk, and other carbohydrates are in the carbohydrate group.

All of the foods in a group have similar amounts of calories and fat. They also have similar amounts of carbohydrates and protein. You can trade or exchange one food for another within a group. The system is easy to follow when you learn the approximate serving size for each group.

A meal plan based on exchange groups lists the number of servings from each group to eat at a meal or snack. You can choose to eat any of the foods within a group. This gives you flexibility in putting your meals together because you have more food choices.

The Food Diary and the Exchange System

A food diary based on the exchange system is pretty simple. When noting the food in your food diary, put a tally mark for each serving eaten next to the name of the food group. At the end of the day, your daily plan should be filled in for each food group.

An example of a meal plan is in the Appendix. When you eat servings from each of the food groups, your meals are nutritionally balanced. To learn more about nutritional balance, read the Food Pyramid section on page 52.

Worksheet 7A: Problem Foods

If you are getting extra calories and fat from foods you eat, this worksheet can help you create a simple plan to limit the amount of fat and calories you eat.

STEP 1. Identify problem foods

Look at the foods you eat. Identify which foods you think contribute the greatest amount of calories.

High-calorie or high-fat foods
1. _____
2. _____
3. _____

STEP 2. Plan low-calorie substitutes

Select at least three lower-calorie items that you can substitute for the problem foods. You can use a calorie/fat counter or book if you are having trouble. Look at how many calories you would save if you made these small changes.

Lower-calorie foods	Calories/fat saved
1. _____	1. _____
2. _____	2. _____
3. _____	3. _____

If you count calories: By making these changes, I plan to save a total of _____ calories.

If you count grams of fat: By making these changes, I plan to save a total of _____ grams of fat.

STEP 3. Take action

At least two times this week, substitute the low-calorie foods that you have selected.

Exchanges—Quick Counting Method

If you know the serving size, you can "guess" how much fat and calories you are eating.

Starches

Serving	1 slice, ½ cup, or 1 oz
Calories	About 80
Fat	0 g

Vegetables

Serving	½ cup cooked or 1 cup raw
Calories	About 25
Fat	0 g

Milk

Serving	8 oz of skim or low-fat milk or 8 oz nonfat or low-fat yogurt
Calories	Skim milk = 90
	Low-fat milk = 120
	Nonfat yogurt = 90
	Low-fat yogurt = 120
Fat	Skim milk or nonfat yogurt = 0 g
	Low-fat milk or yogurt = 1–2 g

Fruit

Serving	1 medium fruit, ½ cup canned (unsweetened), or ½ cup juice
Calories	about 60 (may vary)
Fat	0 g

Meat and Substitutes

Serving	1 oz cooked meat, eggs, fish, or poultry
Calories	Very lean: 35
	Lean or low fat: 55
	Medium fat: 75
	High fat: 100
Fat	Very lean: 0–1 g
	Lean or low fat: 3 g
	Medium fat: 5 g
	High fat: 8 g

Fat

Serving   1 tsp margarine or cooking oils; 1 Tbsp regular salad dressing
Calories   About 45
Fat   5 g

Free Foods

Serving   Unlimited
Calories   Less than 20
Fat   0 g

Worksheet 7B: Using the Exchange System

Are you familiar with the exchange system? Here is an opportunity to check. How would you identify each food in the following meal using the exchange system? If you are confused, go back to the Quick Counting section on page 50, or check the lists on pages 53–55.

For example, if for dinner you ate

- 1 cup spaghetti
- 2 meatballs weighing 1 oz each
- 1 cup salad
- 2 tsp Russian dressing
- 12 oz unsweetened iced tea

How would you record this meal in your food diary? Fill in Monday's column. The answers are on page 56.

Food groups	Plan	Mon	Tue	Wed	Thu	Fri	Sat	Sun
Starches	5							
Meats	4							
Vegetables	3							
Fruits	2							
Milks								
Fats	3							

The Food Pyramid

The food pyramid can help you choose foods for a healthy diet. The chart below will give you a good idea about how much food to eat each day. The size of the section and its location on the pyramid remind you how much to eat of each food group. Some pyramid serving sizes are different from exchange servings. If you use the pyramid, be sure to eat the correct serving size.

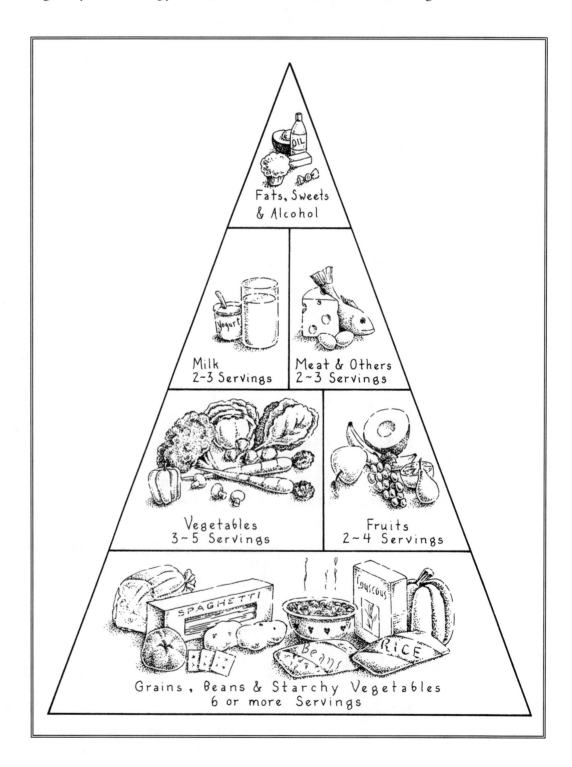

Recommended Pyramid Servings for Your Plan*

1200 calories	1500 calories	1800 calories
6 starches	7 starches	9 starches
3 fruits	3 fruits	3 fruits
2 (4 oz meat or substitute)	2 (5 oz meat or substitute)	2 (6 oz meat or substitute)
3 vegetables	3 vegetables	4 vegetables
2–5 fats	4–9 fats	5–11 fats
2 milks	2–3 milks	2–3 milks
+ free food	+ free food	+ free food

*from *Diabetes Meal Planning Made Easy*, p. 147.

Exchange Serving Sizes

Here are examples of servings in each exchange food group. Measure until you can correctly eyeball serving sizes.

Starch (about ½ cup/serving)

- 1 slice bread
- ¾ cup cold breakfast cereal
- ½ cup cooked cereal (oatmeal)
- ½ cup pasta or ⅓ cup rice
- ⅓ cup beans (chickpeas, lentils, kidney beans)
- 1 starchy vegetable (one 6-inch corn cob, 1 small or ½ cup mashed potato)

Meats and substitutes (per oz)—Low fat

- All fresh or frozen fish with no added fat (no cream or oily sauces, not fried)
- Chicken or turkey breast cooked without the skin
- London broil
- Sirloin
- Flank steak
- Pork tenderloin
- Fresh ham
- Boiled ham (canned or cured)
- Any nonfat cheeses
- Low-fat cottage cheeses
- Egg white
- Shellfish
- Tuna, herring, and sardines in water

Meats and substitutes (per oz)—Medium fat

- Chicken or turkey with skin
- Most beef products—ground beef, roast, steak, meatloaf, and veal
- Porkchops, pork loin roast, pork cutlets
- Lamb chops, leg and roast
- Tuna in oil, rinsed and drained
- Canned salmon
- Liver, heart, kidney, and sweetbreads
- Skim, part-skim cheeses (ricotta, mozzarella, other diet cheeses)
- Whole eggs
- Tofu

Meats and substitutes (per oz)—High fat

- Most USDA prime cuts of meat, such as ribs, corned beef
- All fried fish and fish products
- Luncheon meats
- Frankfurters
- Regular cheeses (American, blue, cheddar, Monterey Jack, Swiss)
- Peanut butter (1 Tbsp)

Fats (usually 1 tsp/serving)

- Butter, margarine, oil, or mayonnaise
- Cream cheese
- Nuts or seeds
- 2 Tbsp sour cream, light cream, nondairy creamer, reduced-fat cream cheese
- 1 slice bacon
- 1 Tbsp regular salad dressing

Vegetables (1 cup raw, ½ cup cooked)

- Asparagus
- Beans (green, wax)
- Beets
- Broccoli
- Brussels sprouts
- Cabbage
- Carrots
- Cauliflower
- Green pepper
- Mushrooms (cooked)
- Onions
- Sauerkraut
- Spinach
- Tomatoes
- Turnips

Fruits
- Apple (2 inch diameter), 1
- Apricot (½ cup)
- Banana (9 inches)
- Cantaloupe (cubed 1 cup)
- Cherries (½ cup)
- Grapefruit (medium)
- ½ cup grapes
- ½ orange
- Peach
- Pear
- Pineapple (⅓ cup)
- Raspberries (1 cup)
- Strawberries (1¼ cups)
- Watermelon (1¼ cups)
- Juices (⅓ to ½ cup)

Milk (1 cup)
- Skim milk and low-fat yogurt

Free Food
- Horseradish
- Mustard
- Nonfat salad dressing
- Nonfat salsa
- Celery
- Cucumbers
- Peppers
- Cranberries
- Rhubarb
- Most vegetables

Free Drinks
- Tea (without milk)
- Coffee (without milk)
- Sugar-free soft drinks
- Nonfat bouillon

Free Extras
- Garlic
- Herbs
- Soy sauce
- Lime or lemon
- All seasonings and spices

Answers to **Worksheet 7B: Using the Exchange System** from page 51

Your food diary would look like:

Food groups	Plan	Mon	Tue	Wed	Thu	Fri	Sat	Sun
Starches		//						
Meats		//						
Vegetables		/						
Fruits		/						
Milks								
Fats		/						

- If you had 1 cup of spaghetti, you would put two tally marks in for the starch. (1 starch exchange = ½ cup)
- After you weighed your meat ball and found that they were 1 ounce, you would put two tally marks in the meat group. If they were larger, you should mark more.
- If the meat balls were fried, then you would check a teaspoon of fat for each meatball. That would be two teaspoons of fat.
- For one cup of salad you would mark 1 vegetable in the vegetable tally column.
- One tablespoon of regular Russian salad dressing equals 1 serving of fat, so you would put one tally mark in the fat group.
- If your iced tea was unsweetened or diet, you do not have to do anything. If it was sweetened, you would have to give up some fruit or starch for it. That might not be a very good trade or exchange (1 tsp sugar = ½ fruit).

CHAPTER EIGHT

Reducing Fat and Calories at the Table

This chapter helps you prevent extra fat and calories from derailing your good intentions to lose weight. There are basic strategies you can follow:

- Stop eating the foods that are high in fat and calories.
- Eat the food less often.
- Change the recipe by reducing the fat and calories.
- Substitute foods that are lower in fat.

Focus on Your Food: The 20-Minute Rule

Did you know that it takes about 20 minutes for your stomach to send a signal to your brain that it is full? Try to time yourself during meals. If you eat an entire meal in 10 to 15 minutes, you are eating too quickly.

Here is how to follow the 20-minute rule.

- If you want a second helping of food, always wait 20 minutes. This way, you give your body time to respond.

- Before having dessert, leave the table for a few minutes. Give your body some time to process the food you just ate. You may find that you feel too full for dessert.

Eat your meals slowly. Take time to savor the foods. It is also best to finish chewing the last bite before eating the next one. Relax. Mealtime should be your time.

- Count the number of times you chew each bite. Go for 25 or more.
- Divide the food on your plate in half, eat the first half, and sit for 3 minutes before eating the second half.
- Eat meals only when sitting down.
- Avoid eating while watching television, reading, or working. These types of activities do not allow you to focus on your food.

Reducing Fat and Calories in Your Cooking

Eliminating some fat from your meal plan makes your meals healthier and brings you one step closer to your weight-management goals. Remember that fat has twice as many calories as protein or carbohydrate. You learn more about ways of eliminating high-fat items later in the chapter.

> Every time you eliminate a tablespoon of fat from your meal, you save 100 calories.

Think about your favorite foods. You can reduce fat by 25% or more in their recipes and still retain the taste and texture of the food. You may need to add more liquid to the recipe.

Many high-fat recipes are high in calories not only because of fat but also because of sweeteners such as sugar. For example, ½ cup of sugar is almost 400 calories. Sugar can be reduced by 25 or 35% in baking, and your baked goods will still be crisp and tasty.

You do not have to give up all the foods you like to eat. Just be aware of the serving sizes. A smaller serving will give you the taste you enjoy but not as many of the calories.

Substituting an Ingredient

To substitute an ingredient in your recipes, you need to determine how it affects appearance, taste, and texture. In some cases, you can find a healthy substitute that will work. In other cases, you cannot.

You can learn how to alter your recipes without feeling you are missing out on the foods that you enjoy. For example, if you use extra-lean ground beef instead of regular ground round, you will save about 150 calories and 15 grams of fat for each 3-oz serving. If you use ½ cup nonfat plain yogurt instead of ½ cup regular sour cream, you save 60 calories and 12 grams of fat.

Worksheet 8A: Recipe Makeover Exercise

This exercise can help you identify high-fat ingredients in a recipe and choose substitutes for them. Read the following recipe, then choose ingredients that could be substituted to lower the fat and calories.

Nana Maria's Original Lasagna
2 cups ricotta cheese
1 26 oz jar spaghetti sauce
8 or 9 lasagna noodles cooked according to package directions
½ lb Italian sausage, sliced into ½-inch rounds
½ lb ground round, browned, crumbled, and drained
2½ cups shredded mozzarella cheese
Oregano, garlic, or black pepper for taste

What substitutions would you make for this recipe to make it lower in fat and calories?

High-fat ingredients   Lower-fat substitutes

_____   _____
_____   _____
_____   _____

Look at the answer key on page 63 to see whether the foods you substituted matched ours.

Approaching Food Habits in a New Way

The following section can help you come closer to your weight-loss goals. It gives you suggestions for lowering fats and calories in your meals. You already may be familiar with some of these suggestions. Now is a great time to put them to action! Begin gradually. We recommend you choose five suggestions to focus on each week. Change is a process, so do not be discouraged if you find it difficult at first. Keep going...you can do it!

Poultry
1. If you usually eat chicken with skin on it, *try removing the skin.*
2. If you fry chicken or turkey in oil, *try baking, broiling, or poaching instead.*

Meat
1. If you usually add sausage or other meat to flavor your sauces, *try to use seasonings such as garlic, fennel, or sage to replace the sausage.*
2. If you often consume large portions of meat, *try to eat smaller portions of meat and increase the portions of rice, pasta, or vegetables.*
3. If you usually choose high-fat cuts of meat, *try to use leaner cuts of meat or choose poultry instead.*
4. If you fry your meat in oil, *try baking, broiling, or grilling instead of frying.*
5. If you eat red meat without trimming the fat, *try trimming visible fat from your meats.*

Fish & Eggs
1. If you eat tuna packed in oil, *try using water-packed tuna, or rinse oil-packed tuna before using it.*
2. If you eat seafood that is high in fat and calories, such as fried shrimp, *try baking or broiling the fish or seafood.*
3. If you have more than 3 whole eggs a week, including eggs used in baking and breaded foods, *try eating 2 egg whites instead of a whole egg, or reduce the number of eggs you have each week.*

Milk & Cheese
1. If you usually drink whole milk or use whole milk in baking, *use skim milk or low-fat (1%) milk instead of whole milk whenever possible.*
2. If you eat yogurt made from whole milk, *try fat-free or low-fat yogurt.*
3. If you have premium ice cream for dessert, *try low-calorie frozen yogurt or reduced-fat ice cream.*
4. If you eat cheese made from whole milk, *try fat-free, low-fat, or low-calorie cheeses.*
5. If you eat regular cream cheese, *try fat-free or low-fat cream cheese.*

Fruits

1. If you eat fruits canned in heavy syrup, *try eating fresh fruit or fruit canned in natural juices.*
2. If you rarely eat fresh fruit, *try eating fresh fruits several times a week.*
3. If you rarely or never have fresh fruits to replace high-calorie snacks, *try eating fresh fruits during snack times.*
4. If you only have fruits when prepared in cakes and pies, *try to add more of a variety to your meal plan by having fresh fruits and fruit juices several days a week.*

Salads & Vegetables

1. If you put thick, rich dressings on your salads, *try low-fat and reduced-calorie dressings, salsa, or seasonings instead.*
2. If you add luncheon meats and cheeses to your salads (as in chef salad), *try choosing luncheon meats and cheeses lower in fat, and add more vegetables to your salads.*
3. If you eat very few vegetables daily, *try adding more vegetables to your meal plan by mixing them with your meat, poultry, fish, or grain dishes.*

Baked Foods

Baked and snack foods are generally filled with fat and calories, but you do not have to give up snacking.

1. If you eat high-fat baked goods, *try baking your own instead of buying baked goods.*
2. If you add whole milk to recipes, *try substituting low-fat or skim milk.*
3. If you place glaze or canned icing on cakes, *try adding low-calorie glaze or low-fat canned icing on cakes.*
4. If you usually prepare two-crust pies, *try a one-crust pie.*
5. If you make creamed pie fillings, *try skim milk, low-fat ricotta cheese, or low-fat yogurt with gelatin topping.*
6. If you use solid baking chocolate in your recipes, *try unsweetened cocoa powder.*

Snack Foods

1. If you consume high-fat dips and snacks, *try nonfat or low-fat dip and salsa.*
2. If you eat regular potato chips, corn chips, and taco chips, *try air-popped "lite" popcorn, pretzels, or baked corn and potato chips.*
3. If you tend to eat too many cookies at one time, *try not to eat from the package. Set aside the number of cookies you'll eat at one time and put the package away.*

Fats

1. If you add butter to your meals, *try using low-fat jams or jellies, low-fat yogurt, nonfat sour cream, whipped butter, or tub margarine. In baking, try applesauce, fruit, or other low-fat spreads.*
2. If you add thick sauces or gravy to meat or poultry, *try adding flavor with lemon juice, wine, herbs, and other low-fat seasonings.*

3. If you usually use regular mayonnaise, *try using reduced-fat mayonnaise or nonfat imitation salad dressings. Mix with plain nonfat yogurt.*
4. If you add sour cream to your recipes, *try using nonfat sour cream or nonfat yogurt.*

Eliminating High-Fat Items

1. If you tend to eat a lot of meat with your meals, *try choosing less fatty but flavorful cuts of meat. Also try mixing vegetables and grains in your meals, and cut back on your portions of meat.*
2. If you have a buttered roll with your meal, *remove the roll, or replace it with a salad. You can also have the roll without butter, or serve yourself a smaller serving of bread.*
3. If you add extras like cheese, dressings, or gravy to food, *try to cut back on the extras by reducing your portions or using a reduced-fat or nonfat substitute.*
4. If you tend to overeat during the main course, *try having a salad before, and reduce your serving of the main course to feel satisfied without extra fat and calories.*

Adding or Increasing Flavor

Many people complain that food tastes bland and does not look appetizing when ingredients are substituted in recipes. You can add flavorful ingredients that will decrease fat and calories and still taste terrific.

Ways to Increase Flavor

1. Increase garlic, herbs, and other spices.
2. Add more vegetables to soups, stews, and sauces.
3. Add hot sauces, salsa, mustard, or horseradish.
4. Create your own spices to flavor your foods.
5. Add low-sodium chicken or beef bouillon granules.

Changing a Cooking Technique

Changing a cooking technique is another way to keep food low in fat without sacrificing taste. Here are some ways you can reduce fat and calories in your meal.

Baking

1. Bake meatballs instead of browning them in a frying pan with oil.
2. When baking foods in a sauce, skip the sautéing step of the recipe.
3. To increase moisture, spray breaded meat with nonfat cooking spray before baking it.

Sautéing

1. To cut down on the fat in sautéing, spray with nonfat cooking spray or wipe the pan with a paper towel dipped in oil.
2. Use a nonstick frying pan to lightly sauté meats and vegetables.

Broiling or Grilling

1. Pan broil in a nonstick pan instead of frying.
2. Barbecue over an electric or gas grill to reduce fat in your cooking.
3. To keep foods moist when grilling, spray with a nonstick spray before cooking.

Other Methods

1. Refrigerate stew and soup before serving. The fat will accumulate on top, and you can remove it before serving
2. Use a paper towel to absorb fat from food.
3. Use a slotted spoon or spatula to remove fat from the pan.
4. Broil meats instead of frying them.

Low-fat versions of your favorite foods may not taste the same as the higher-fat versions. If you are cooking for a large family, consider ways you can satisfy your family's preferences and your new eating style. For example, if the members of your family object to drinking skim milk, try 1% or 2% milk. Although it is higher in fat and calories, it may be a reasonable compromise.

Never feel that everything you eat must be low in fat and calories. Eating only foods low in fat and calories is the ideal, but most people don't eat that way. Make wise decisions that fit into the meal plan you have chosen.

Recipe Makeover Answers

If your substitutions are different from ours, they may still be good ones. Check your fat and calorie count book to make sure your choices are really lower in fat and calories. Here are our suggestions.

1. Use low-fat or nonfat cottage cheese or part-skim or nonfat ricotta instead of whole-milk ricotta.
2. Use a low-fat or nonfat spaghetti sauce.
3. Leave out the sausage, and season with fennel seeds.
4. Substitute ground turkey and/or a can of beans for the ground meat and sausage.
5. Omit all meat and use more vegetables such as zucchini.
6. Use part-skim mozzarella or low-fat or nonfat Monterey Jack cheese.

■

Reading Food Labels

Food labels provide a rich source of information about the calorie, fat, and nutrition content of your favorite foods. Reading food labels can help you make good food choices.

New Label Laws

In 1993, new label laws were required by the U.S. Food and Drug Administration (FDA). Food labels give information about the fat, cholesterol, carbohydrate, protein, and vitamin and mineral content of foods. Similar foods have similar serving sizes so you can compare them more easily. We discuss these features in the sections that follow.

Using food-label information can help you

- find the most nutritious foods
- compare ingredients and cost
- make choices using calorie and fat information
- choose foods low in total fat, saturated fat, and cholesterol

The following words often appear on food labels:

- Serving size
- Cholesterol
- Fat
- Carbohydrates
- Percent daily values

Finding Calorie and Fat Information

The food label is one of the best sources of fat and calorie information for a particular food. Food labels are usually a more reliable source of fat and calorie information than calorie books, because the information is for the specific product.

The most important thing to remember when looking at information on food labels is to look at the serving size. Two similar products, regardless of the brand name, should have an equal serving size so you can compare the products.

Allison's Cookie Deluxe
Serving size—3 cookies
Calories—200
Fat—9 grams

Arlene's Cocoa Mania Cookie
Serving size—3 cookies
Calories—150
Fat—5 grams

For example, the labels of the two brands of chocolate chip cookies above should give the same serving size (3 cookies) and nutritional information for that product (200 calories, 9 grams of fat for one brand; 150 calories, 5 grams of fat for the other) so you can make a choice between them.

You will find that the serving size is much smaller than most people eat in some cases. Weighing and measuring your food is the only way to be sure of the size of your serving.

Calories and Food Labels

Food labels list the total number of calories per serving and calories from fat. Counting total calories can help you manage your weight, when you stay within a certain calorie range for the day.

Fat Substitutes and Food Labels

Food labels give the fat content in foods. Fat has twice as many calories as protein and carbohydrate, so cutting back on fat saves you calories and can help you lose weight. The amount of fat in foods is listed in grams (g). By counting the fat grams, you can budget how much fat you eat. Keep in mind that the number of fat grams is listed per serving. If you eat more than one serving, remember to add the total fat grams you ate.

There are several fat substitutes on the market that are used as ingredients for baked goods, snacks, and other products. They may not be as low in calories as you might expect. Be aware that eating large quantities of some fat substitutes may cause stomach and digestive upsets. Fat substitutes that are made of carbohydrate will affect your blood sugar level.

The Fat and Calorie Connection

Some people limit fat by choosing only foods that have 30% (or less) calories from fat. However, some of your favorite foods, such as salad dressing and ice cream, have a high percentage of fat. You can balance them by eating low-fat foods at your other meals that day. Fruits, vegetables, and grains have almost no fat. You figure the percentage of calories from fat for the whole day, not for one food. To do this you add up the fat grams in all the foods that you eat in one day and the calories, and follow the steps on page 67.

Check the label! You can check if a food has less than 30% calories from fat.

Nutrition Facts	
Serving size	1 Tbsp
Calories per serving	30
Calories from fat	25
Saturated fat	2 g
Cholesterol	0 mg

The label tells you the total number of calories and the calories from fat. To find the percentage of calories from fat, divide the calories from fat by the total number of calories, and multiply by 100.

$$\frac{\text{calories from fat}}{\text{total calories}} \times 100 = \text{percentage of calories from fat}$$

Developing Label Smarts

Check out the example of Michelle's Mega-Muffins to see how well you understand label information.

Michelle's Mega-Muffins

Serving size	1 muffin (5 oz)
Calories	500
Calories from fat	135
Fat	15 g

How many grams of fat does this item contain per serving?
Michelle's Mega-Muffins have 15 g fat.

How many calories come from fat?
Michelle's Mega-Muffins have 135 calories from fat.
(15 x 9 (calories per gram of fat) = 135 calories from fat.)

What is the percentage of calories from fat?
Michelle's Mega-Muffins get 27% of their calories from fat.

$$\frac{135 \text{ calories from fat}}{500 \text{ total calories}} = 0.27 \times 100 = 27\%$$

Worksheet 9A: The Salami Example

Answer the following questions about salami. One ounce of salami has 100 calories and 8 g fat.

1. How many calories are there in a 3-oz serving? _____

2. How many grams of fat in a 3-oz serving? _____

3. How many calories from fat are in a 3-oz serving? _____

4. What is the percentage of total calories from fat in a 3-oz serving? _____

Answers

1. 100 calories per oz x 3 oz = 300 calories

2. 8 g fat x 3 oz = 24 g fat

3. 24 g fat x 9 calories = 216 calories from fat

4. $\dfrac{216 \text{ calories from fat}}{300 \text{ calories}}$ = 72 x 100 = 72%

Percent Daily Values

Percent daily values (% DV) are also listed on food labels. These are based on the recommended amounts you should eat of the nutrients such as protein, carbohydrate, and fat. Each day (or over a few days), you should get close to 100% of each of these nutrients. No single food has 100% of all the nutrients. That's why the label tells you how much of each you are getting. You add up the amounts you get from each food to find your daily total for each nutrient.

Percent daily values on the label are for a 2000-calorie diet. If you do not eat 2000 calories a day, you need to determine your own nutrient needs for fat, saturated fat, carbohydrates, fiber, and protein. An RD can help you do this. Daily values for cholesterol, sodium, minerals, and vitamins stay the same for all calorie levels.

Percent daily values are based on a 2000-calorie diet

A rule of thumb: If one serving of a food contains more than 20% of a nutrient, pay attention to it. If it has less than 5%, it adds very little to your daily total.

You can figure out your daily value needs by multiplying the 2000-calorie numbers by the factor in the chart below.

Calories	Factors
1200	1.6
1500	1.3
1800	1.1

For example, the food label on a container of cream cheese says that one serving provides 17% of the daily value of fat (for a 2000-calorie diet). If you are on an 1800-calorie diet, you would multiply 17% x 1.1 = 19%. One serving of cream cheese would provide 19% of *your* daily value for fat.

For a 1500-calorie diet, you would multiply 17% x 1.3 = 22%, so one serving would provide 22% of your daily value.

For a 1200-calorie diet, 17% x 1.6 = 27%, so one serving would provide 27% of your daily value.

The label on a can of regular soda says that one serving provides 14% of the daily value for carbohydrates (for a 2000-calorie diet). For an 1800-calorie diet, 14% x 1.1 = 15%, so one serving of soda provides 15% of your daily value for carbohydrates.

For a 1500-calorie diet, 14% x 1.3 = 18%, so one serving of soda provides 18% of your daily value for carbohydrates.

For a 1200-calorie diet, 14% x 1.6 = 22%, so one serving of the soda provides 22% of your daily value for carbohydrates. That's more than 20%, so you'll need to decide if you would rather substitute a diet soda or tea for this regular soda. You may want to get your carbohydrates from another, more nutritious food.

Now that you are somewhat familiar with daily values, you might try this example. A label on a frozen dinner says that it provides 9% of the daily value of fat for a 2000-calorie diet. What would the percent daily values be for a 1200-, 1500-, and 1800-calorie meal plan?

Calories	Multiply by	% Daily value for fat
1200	1.6	_____
1500	1.3	_____
1800	1.1	_____

Answers to this question are on page 75.

You can use percent daily values to compare products.

Nutrition Claims

Now look at this label for light mayonnaise.

Nutrition Facts	
Serving size	1 Tbsp
Calories per serving	30
Calories from fat	25
Saturated fat	2 g
Cholesterol	0 mg

Is *low in cholesterol* the same as *low in fat?* ❑ Yes ❑ No ❑ Don't know

Is this product low in fat? ❑ Yes ❑ No ❑ Don't know

The answer to the first question is no. Do not be misled by bold print saying cholesterol-free. If 25 of the 30 calories in this product come from fat, then about 83% of the calories (25 divided by 30 x 100) are from fat. In addition, there are 2 g of saturated fat (18 calories). If you do the math, you find that 18 calories from saturated fat / 30 total calories = 60% of this product contains saturated fat. Even if a product claims to be low in cholesterol, it can still be high in fat.

If the regular version of this product contains 60 calories per 1 Tbsp serving and 50 of those calories are from fat, the "light" product may be a good choice. You would be getting less fat per serving, so the don't know answer is correct for the second question.

Food labels may be fooling you and you don't even know it.

Besides giving nutritional information, food labels make claims about the product. The label laws of 1993 helped control what manufacturers can claim about their products. The following list of common claims can help you avoid being fooled by claims on the label.

1993 FDA Label Laws for Fat-Related Nutrition Claims

- **Extra lean:** A food labeled **extra lean** contains less than 5 g fat, 2 g saturated fat, and 95 mg cholesterol per 100 g food.
- **Good source of:** A product that is a **good source of** something provides between 10 and 19% of the daily value for that nutrient per serving.
- **High in:** A food that is **high in** something contains 20% or more of the daily value for the nutrient.
- **Lean:** A food that is labeled **lean** has less than 10 g fat, 4 g saturated fat, and 95 mg cholesterol per serving.
- **Light:** A "light" food has ½ the fat and ⅓ fewer calories than a traditionally prepared food item. **Light** can also be used to describe an aspect of the food. For example, a creamy cheese cake is light.
- **Low cholesterol:** Foods low in cholesterol contain no more than 20 mg cholesterol per serving (about 60 mg in a 10-oz main dish or meal).
- **Low in saturated fat:** This means that the product has 1 g or less saturated fat per serving.
- **Low in fat:** Low in fat means at least half of the fat has been removed, and the calories have been cut by ⅓.
- **Reduced:** Also referred to as "less" or "fewer," a reduced product contains 25% less of that nutrient.

Organic Foods

The word *organic* is added to more and more food labels and foods at the supermarket. What does it mean? *Organic foods* are foods grown without the use of pesticides. Because organic growers try to select crops on the basis of taste rather than the way they respond to pesticides, most people think organic foods taste better. Food labeled *certified organic* means that the grocery store can certify that the food was organically grown. The consumer can ask for papers tracing the grower and the location of the organic farm.

Quantity of Ingredients

Manufacturers must list ingredients in the order of their quantity in the product. The ingredient present in the largest amount comes first, the ingredient in the second-largest amount comes second, and the ingredient present in the smallest quantity is listed last. The first three ingredients make up the bulk of the product. Look at the following example.

Spaghetti Sauce A

Ingredients: tomato sauce, tomatoes in tomato juice, tomato paste, vegetable oil, salt, dehydrated onion, imported romano cheese, basil, dehydrated garlic, oregano, black pepper, bay leaf

---

Spaghetti Sauce B

Ingredients: tomatoes, sweeteners, soybean oil, salt, olive oil, spices, garlic powder, natural flavors, dried onions, parsley, lemon juice concentrate

---

Which spaghetti sauce is the best nutritional value? ❏ Sauce A ❏ Sauce B

Spaghetti Sauce A is the best because it lists tomatoes (in one form or another) as the first three ingredients. Spaghetti Sauce B lists tomatoes, sweeteners, and soybean oil as its first three ingredients. Sauce A provides more real tomatoes and fewer sugars (think calories) and fillers than sauce B.

Quality of Ingredients

Sugar

Sugar is often listed as a primary ingredient and makes up the bulk of certain foods. Sugar, as you know, is often found in cakes, cookies, pies, and candy. It is also hidden in foods where you would not expect to find it. If sugar is the one of the first three words on the food label, beware! This food may be high in calories and carbohydrate. High sugar foods may also have a lot of fat.

Sugars appear on food labels as

- sugar
- sucrose
- corn syrup
- dextrose
- molasses

- lactose
- honey
- maltose
- carob
- fructose

On labels, *sweeteners* are listed together after the word sweeteners, in descending order of the amount present. The ingredients on a bottle of blueberry jam could be listed as sweeteners (corn syrup, sugar), blueberries, fruit pectin, citric acid.

Fat

Manufacturers often use the words listed below to describe the hidden fats in their products. If you ever see these words, read the food label carefully. You may notice the food is high in fat and calories.

Fats appear on labels as

- diglycerides
- monoglycerides
- oil
- coconut

- butter
- lard
- cream

Saturated Fat

There are several types of fat. One type is usually solid at room temperature and is called **saturated fat.** Saturated fat causes your body to produce more cholesterol. One of the benefits of cutting back on fat, especially saturated fat, is the resulting decrease in your blood cholesterol levels. People get a lot of saturated fat from snack foods such as potato chips and crackers and from desserts such as cookies, cakes, pies, pastries, and ice cream. Saturated fat is often listed on labels as butter, lard, hydrogenated oil, and coconut oil.

Cutting back on saturated fats can also help prevent heart disease and hypertension. People with diabetes have a high risk of developing heart disease, so watching the cholesterol you eat is important. Cholesterol is carried through the bloodstream in the form of lipoproteins—a compound of fats and proteins. High density lipoprotein (HDL) cholesterol is called "good" because it helps prevent cholesterol deposits from attaching to blood vessel walls. The low density lipoproteins (LDL), however, increase the chances of cholesterol being deposited in your blood vessels. Being overweight contributes to many heart disease risk factors such as high blood pressure, high total cholesterol, low HDL cholesterol levels, and high triglycerides.

Polyunsaturated Fat

Another type of fat is **polyunsaturated fat,** which is found in corn and sunflower oils. It is usually a liquid, even when chilled.

Monounsaturated Fat

The third type of fat is usually a liquid and is called **monounsaturated fat.** It is found in olives (olive oil), peanuts, avocados, and canola oil. This is the best type of fat.

Smart Shopper Sam

Sam went to the grocery store to buy cheese. He wanted a low-fat spreadable cheese but had a hard time picking the one with the least calories and fat. He had a choice:

- light cream cheese with 80% calories from fat
- low-fat cottage cheese with 10% calories from fat.

He chose the low-fat cottage cheese. This is how Sam decided. One serving (1/2 cup) of cottage cheese had 90 calories and 1 g fat. One serving of light cream cheese (1 oz) had 70 calories and 6 g fat.

One serving of cottage cheese had 9 calories (1 g fat x 9 calories per g fat) from fat in 90 calories, or 10% fat. One serving of light cream cheese has 54 calories from fat per serving (6 g fat x 9 calories). He did the following calculation

$$\frac{54}{70} = 0.80 \text{ x } 100 = 80\% \text{ fat}$$

Sam picked the lower-fat alternative. He could also have picked a nonfat cream cheese, which is lower in calories (25 calories per oz) with no fat.

Answers for Daily Values for fat

Calories	Multiply by	% Daily value for fat
1200	1.6	15%
1500	1.3	12%
1800	1.1	10%

In this chapter, you
- develop healthy shopping strategies
- learn skills for smart food storage

CHAPTER TEN

Shopping Strategies and Food Storage

Going grocery shopping gives you an opportunity to apply what you know about reading food labels. Shopping strategies and food storage tips help you make healthy food choices.

Shopping Strategies

High-fat foods are the most common source of excess calories in your meal plan. A simple strategy is not to buy them.

Supermarkets are designed to get you to shop on impulse, that is, to purchase as much food as possible. It is no accident that snack foods, soda, and cakes are often at the ends of aisles or at the checkout stand where you will notice them several times during your shopping trip.

The strategies below can make healthy shopping much easier.

1. Do not go shopping when you are hungry—an empty stomach and a full grocery store can lead to impulsive purchases based on hunger rather than healthy choices.

2. Do not go shopping without a list—organize your list according to the categories in the grocery store or the way you walk down the aisles. For example, list all the fruits and vegetables in one place and all the dairy products together in another. Having a shopping list will prevent you from wandering down the aisles wondering what you forgot to buy.

3. Buy foods that you must prepare.
   - Instead of potato chips, buy unpopped popcorn that you can make for yourself in small amounts.
   - Instead of having a ready-made cake in the house for company, buy a cake mix or bake from scratch.
   - Instead of cold cuts, buy tuna in water or lean hamburger that you have to prepare.

4. Do not buy things just because they are on sale or because you have a coupon.
   - Stop and think, Does this fit into my healthy-eating lifestyle?
   - Buy only what is on your shopping list. Your health is more important than saving a few cents on a high-calorie "bargain."

5. Buy foods that are individually portioned instead of in large quantities, even though they cost more.

Controlling your portion sizes will help keep you from eating too many calories and fat grams.

The next time you go to the store, ask yourself how you can boost the nutritional value of your food and keep the calories and fats low. List below any changes you have made or you would consider making in your purchasing patterns. List four foods that you used to eat or now eat that are high in fat and calories. What are some products you could buy that are lower in calories and fat? For example, if you buy lower-fat cheese instead of cuts of meat or whole milk cheeses, write it down.

Instead of	I will buy
1. _____	1. _____
2. _____	2. _____
3. _____	3. _____
4. _____	4. _____

Food Storage

Once you bring your food home, the way you store it can influence when and how much you eat. The following suggestions may make you more conscious of how you store your foods.

1. Put the food away with a plan.
   • Keep higher-calorie foods out of sight or in hard-to-reach places. Keep lower-calorie foods up front and easy to reach.

2. Make food less visible.
   • Keep cookies, crackers, and other snack foods in the pantry rather than on the counter or table.

3. Repackage tempting foods into smaller servings.
   • If you prepare servings ahead of time, you will be less likely to eat an extra serving and increase your calorie and fat gram count.

4. Wash fruits so they are ready to eat. Place some cut vegetables such as carrots and celery in a plastic bag or container in the refrigerator.

CHAPTER **ELEVEN**

Eating Out

Healthy eating does not mean you have to eat at home. You can eat out, but you need to be aware of challenges you may face at a restaurant or a party. This chapter helps you develop strategies for healthy eating when you eat away from home.

Let's begin by looking at some tips you can use in restaurants.

Basic Tips for Eating Out

Tip 1: Have a low-calorie, low-fat snack before you leave home or as an appetizer.

Having a low-calorie snack can take the edge off your appetite. You'll have more control if you are not starving.

Tip 2: Avoid having more than the portion you planned to eat.

Restaurants often serve huge portions—more food than anyone needs. Take half your portion home for another meal, or share your meal with a friend.

Tip 3: Watch for high-calorie beverages.

Drinking high-calorie beverages can add several hundred calories. Fruit punch, fruit juice, and regular soda contain 9 or 10 teaspoons of sugar for a 12-ounce serving and may add 150 calories or more. Avoid using high-calorie beverages like regular soda, juice, or alcohol to quench your thirst. Have ice water, sugar-free soda, seltzer, or unsweetened tea or coffee.

Alcoholic beverages may contain as many calories as desserts. Alcohol has 7 calories per gram (only 2 calories less than a gram of fat). Also, mixers added to the alcohol have calories and/or fat. For example, a 10-ounce Piña Colada, which includes rum, pineapple juice, and coconut milk, has about 475 calories—about the same as a dessert. White wine, dry red wine, wine spritzers, champagne, or light beer have the fewest calories. Foods people usually eat while drinking alcohol are often high in fat and calories. For example, ¼ cup of nuts has 170 calories and 15 grams of fat. The salty items that are frequently served in bars are designed to make you thirsty so that you will order more drinks. Alcohol can stimulate your appetite.

Tip 4: Be wise with dessert.

If there is a high-calorie, high-fat dessert you cannot resist, have a meal low in fat and calories to balance the overall calories and fat you consume. You can also share your dessert with a friend or friends. The carbohydrate in the dessert will raise blood sugar levels.

How to Eat in Social Settings

Social settings make it harder to select healthy foods. Here are three strategies you can follow to help you master these situations.

Strategy 1: Focus on the setting you are in.

Social settings provide a great environment to talk with people, dance, catch up with old friends, and make new ones. Be conscious of what you eat in these settings. When people are preoccupied, they may not realize how much they are eating. Have a small snack before you leave home to take the edge off your appetite.

Strategy 2: Plan some physical activity the day of the event.

Physical activity is a way to take good care of yourself and burn calories. It also can make you calmer when you get to the party.

Strategy 3: Watch where you sit or stand, and use portion control.

Try to avoid sitting or standing near the buffet table and be selective about the foods you eat. Instead of piling food on your plate, only choose one or two items. Limit your intake of high-fat foods. Fill up on fruits and salads.

Strategy 4: Bring a low-fat or low-calorie food to share.

Others may want to join you in eating better.

Worksheet 11A: Take Charge

Think about how each of the following behaviors applies to you.

- If it is something you do now, put a Y in the space to the left of the behavior.
- If it is something you think you can try doing, put a check next to the behavior.
- If the behavior does not apply to you or you are not ready to try it, leave the space blank.

I can or will

_____ Picture myself successfully eating a low-calorie meal.

_____ Ask for salad dressings and sauces to be served on the side.

_____ Ask for skim milk or low-fat milk instead of cream in my coffee.

_____ Ask the waiter to remove high-fat extras such as fried noodles, chips, or butter with the bread served before or with my meal.

_____ Ask for chicken or fish to be cooked in wine, not butter.

_____ Order foods that are naturally low in fat such as chicken, turkey, fish, and veal.

_____ Order from the menu or request foods that are steamed, broiled, roasted, or poached in their own juices or in tomato sauce.

_____ Send back food that was not prepared the low-fat way I expected.

_____ Take half of my portion home for another meal.

_____ Get up from the table before I order dessert.

_____ Say no if other people push me to have extra food.

_____ Avoid sitting next to the bowl of potato chips or the buffet table.

_____ Share dessert with a friend or ask to take half of it home.

_____ Bring some diet soda, seltzer, raw vegetables or other low-calorie and low-fat contributions to a party or potluck dinner.

_____ Drink sugar-free soda and/or use it as a mixer in beverages.

_____ At a restaurant, decide what to order before being influenced by others.

Number of behaviors marked with a Y _____

Number of behaviors marked with a check _____

Total _____

Order From the Menu Carefully

Read the menu carefully to see what options you have for low-fat and low-calorie items. Remember, you can ask to have dishes modified by leaving off sauces or having the sauce on the side. You can also ask about having an item such as fish grilled with lemon instead of butter.

If you order a la carte, you can save calories, fat, and money. In addition, ordering a la carte keeps you from eating items you really don't want. Ordering an appetizer such as shrimp cocktail with a salad as a main course is a great way to add variety to your meal while keeping your portions small and healthy.

Decide what you are going to order before you listen to what other people are ordering. Try to order first to avoid getting tempted by what others choose.

Watch out for high-fat choices. Look for words such as

- au gratin
- gravy
- breaded
- hollandaise
- buttered or buttery
- parmesan
- cheese sauce
- pastry

- creamed, creamy, in cream sauce
- rich
- sautéed
- fried, deep fried, french fried, batter fried, pan fried
- scalloped
- southern style

Look for low-fat choices, shown by words such as

- baked
- poached
- boiled
- roasted

- broiled
- steamed
- grilled
- stir-fried

What Should I Order?

No matter what kind of restaurant you go to, you can make lower-fat choices. Use the following list to make wise choices:

Red Light: High-fat choices	Green Light: Lower-fat choices
Pizza meat toppings olives artichokes double cheese	cheese onions, green peppers, mushrooms, tomatoes, pineapple
Mexican enchiladas chili con queso fried tortillas, tortilla chips sour cream, guacamole crispy tacos taco salad	tortillas (not fried) grilled chicken or beef fajitas soft tacos (corn or flour tortillas) salsa
Chinese and Japanese egg foo young fried chicken, beef, fish fried rice or noodles egg rolls fried wontons tempura sweet and sour dishes	stir-fried chicken in a little oil stir-fried vegetables in a little oil steamed rice teriyaki chicken or fish soup

Red Light: High-fat choices	Green Light: Lower-fat choices
Italian sausage lasagna, manicotti, other pasta dishes with cheese or cream fried or breaded dishes (like veal or eggplant parmesan) olives regular Italian dressing	spaghetti with meatless tomato sauce minestrone soup tossed salad with low-fat dressing, no cheese or olives linguini with red clam sauce mussels marinara veal with peppers
Seafood fried fish fried vegetables french fries hush puppies cole slaw	broiled, baked or boiled seafood with lemon plain baked potato tossed salad with low-fat dressing, no cheese or olives
Steak houses steak fried chicken or fish onion rings and other fried vegetables french fries	shrimp cocktail broiled chicken or fish plain baked potato tossed salad with low-fat dressing, no cheese or olives
Fast food cheeseburgers whole-milk milkshakes fried fish and chicken french fries mayonnaise-based sauce cole slaw	broiled or baked chicken broiled extra-lean burgers tossed salad with low-fat dressing, no cheese or olives baked potatoes

You cannot always judge an item by the way it is described on the menu. Ask for a copy of the nutrition information at your favorite fast-food place to make the best choice. Most fast-food restaurants are part of a chain, and product information can be obtained from their headquarters if it is not available locally.

Making healthy food choices in social settings or restaurants is possible. You can follow your plan and still enjoy the good things in life. Go out and enjoy the party!

FITNESS &
HEALTH

CHAPTER **TWELVE**

In this chapter, you learn
- how physical fitness can affect heart disease, diabetes, gallbladder disease, and arthritis
- about the set-point theory

Health Benefits of Physical Activity

The human body is made for physical activity. A fit body works better in all ways. Physical activity is one of the most enjoyable parts of a healthy lifestyle. It lowers your risk of getting some conditions and diseases. Fitness and weight loss can slow the progress of heart disease, high blood pressure, diabetes, gallbladder disease, and arthritis. Overweight people who are fit are healthier than thin, inactive people. Regardless of whether you are at your weight goal, you can be reaping the health benefits of fitness today. Research also shows that people who exercise as well as count calories lose weight and keep it off. Exercise is the secret ingredient to successful weight loss.

Preventing Disease

Heart Disease

The heart must work harder when you are overweight. Because you need an extra mile of blood vessels for each pound of fat you have, the extra work by your heart can result in high blood pressure (hypertension). Losing even a small amount of weight can decrease your heart's work and the force it must exert. A physically fit heart will pump more efficiently, too. This is discussed in more detail in chapter 13.

Diabetes

The food you eat is converted to glucose, a sugar that flows through your blood (blood sugar). Insulin is produced by your pancreas to help the blood glucose get into the cells where it is used as energy. When you are heavy, your body needs more insulin to "unlock" the cells because the cells are resistant to insulin. This can lead to diabetes. Using a fitness plan to lose weight can reduce the amount of insulin you need. Regular exercise can also help your body use insulin more efficiently and keep your blood glucose at normal levels.

In addition, physical activity can lower your blood sugar levels for hours afterward. If you exercise vigorously and have diabetes, monitor your blood sugar levels to see how it changes. You may need to alter your meal plan or medication to keep it from going too low. Ask your doctor or diabetes educator for help with this.

Caution! If you try to get in shape too quickly, you can do more harm to your body than good. Use the worksheet on page 94 to determine whether you need a checkup before beginning a fitness program. Also, if you have been exercising at a moderate pace for more than one hour, you need to eat something during or right after your workout to avoid hypoglycemia (very low blood sugar levels.)

Gallbladder Disease

Gallstones and gallbladder disease are linked to a high-fat diet and increased weight. Participating in physical activity can lower your weight and help control gallbladder problems.

Arthritis

Being overweight puts extra stress on your joints, which can make arthritis and inflammation of your joints worse. Physical fitness can help you lose excess weight and lighten the stress on your joints. Following a fitness plan can also help you become more flexible and make it easier for your joints to move. Exercising in water is often more effective and less painful. If your joints swell or you have a lot of pain after exercising, tell your doctor.

Set-Point Theory

The set-point theory can help explain why some people have difficulty losing weight. The set point is the level of weight your body wants to maintain. Your body stays at its set point by adjusting your metabolic rate. When your body weight falls below the set point, your metabolism slows down so that your weight returns to the set point.

Exercise is the primary method for adjusting your set point. Exercise can actually speed up your metabolism and change the set point. Muscles that are fit burn calories even when they are at rest.

Set-Point Paul

Let's look at Paul, whose set point is between 165 and 175 pounds. When Paul's weight goes below 165 pounds, his metabolism slows down so that it burns fewer calories. When his weight goes above 175 pounds, his metabolism quickens so that it burns calories faster. To change his set point to 150 pounds, Paul must make sure to include physical activity in his daily life and to exercise on a regular basis.

Do you know what your set point is?

CHAPTER **THIRTEEN**

Beginning with Fitness Basics

In this chapter, we explore the basics of engaging in physical fitness and dispel some of the myths you often hear.

Spot Reducing Is Impossible

When we lose weight, we lose it all over—from the face, arms, trunk, buttocks, hips, and thighs. Everyone's body is different. Yet we all imagine ideal bodies and how we would like to look. If putting on fat around the middle or in hips and thighs runs in your family, losing weight will not change your basic shape. Do not be discouraged! You may not be able to create the figure of a 17-year old, but you can look fabulous and shine in your own way.

Men and women often have different concerns about how their bodies look and where their fat is distributed. There is nothing you can do to get rid of fat in a specific area—spot reducing does not work—but there are things you can do to fight fat-distribution problems.

The human body's fat consistency is similar to butter. Take a pound of butter and hold it against your belly. It is substantial. If you can, hold 5 pounds against yourself. It is quite an impressive amount of bulk. When you lose 1 pound or 5 pounds, it is the same as taking off the pound of butter you held against your midsection.

Fighting Cellulite or a Bulging Middle

Women and Fat Distribution

Women tend to have a pear-shaped body. That is, they tend to be slimmer on top and carry most of their weight at their hips and thighs. Along with this distribution of fat often comes cellulite. Cellulite is a lumpy accumulation of fat just below the skin. There are no specific exercises that you can do to target the cellulite. Taking walks daily, doing some stretches, and lifting light weights twice a week is the way to combat this condition.

Men and Fat Distribution

Men often have an apple-shaped body. They carry the majority of fat around the waist. A potbelly can put men (and some women) at risk for developing cardiovascular disease. It is often the target of intense but unsuccessful spot reducing.

There are two things you *can* do:

1. Control your weight through regular aerobic exercise and a low-fat, low-calorie diet.
2. Tone the muscles in the problem areas. Aerobic exercise and strength training with weights works and tones those muscles.

A final note: People who tend to carry the majority of their weight around their waist are at a greater risk for developing cardiovascular disease and diabetes. This is especially true for women.

Worksheet 13A: Seeing Your Doctor

Fill out this questionnaire. If you check yes after any of these questions, see your doctor *before* beginning a fitness program.

1. Has a doctor ever said you had heart trouble? ❑ Yes ❑ No
2. Do you have angina pectoris? ❑ Yes ❑ No
3. Have you ever taken medication for your heart? ❑ Yes ❑ No
4. Do you have a history of heart disease including heart attack, valve disease, congestive heart failure, myocarditis, or any other heart disease treated by a physician? ❑ Yes ❑ No
5. Have you ever had an electrocardiogram (ECG)? ❑ Yes ❑ No
6. Have you ever had an ECG taken while you were exercising that was not normal? ❑ Yes ❑ No
7. Do you have or have you ever had a heart murmur? ❑ Yes ❑ No
8. Have you ever had a stroke? ❑ Yes ❑ No
9. Have you ever had any irregular heart action or palpitations? ❑ Yes ❑ No
10. Have you ever had chest pain or a squeezing feeling in the chest that was brought on by exercising, walking, or any other physical or sexual activity? ❑ Yes ❑ No
11. If you climb a few flights of stairs fairly rapidly, do you have a tightness or pressing pain in your chest? ❑ Yes ❑ No
12. Do you have diabetes, or have you had high blood sugar, or sugar in the urine? ❑ Yes ❑ No
13. Do you have high blood pressure that is poorly controlled (resting blood pressure greater than 160 mmHg systolic or 100 mmHg diastolic)? ❑ Yes ❑ No
14. In your family has more than one person had a heart attack or heart trouble before age 60 years? ❑ Yes ❑ No
15. Do you have a high blood cholesterol level? ❑ Yes ❑ No
16. Do you smoke more than a pack and a half of cigarettes per day? ❑ Yes ❑ No
17. Do you have any acute infectious disease (cold, flu, virus, etc.)? ❑ Yes ❑ No
18. Are you more than 20 pounds overweight? ❑ Yes ❑ No
19. Do you suffer from any chronic illness? ❑ Yes ❑ No
20. Do you have asthma, emphysema, or another lung condition? ❑ Yes ❑ No
22. Do you become short of breath easier than other people? ❑ Yes ❑ No
23. Do you often get cramps in your legs if you walk several blocks? ❑ Yes ❑ No
24. Have you ever had or do you have phlebitis? ❑ Yes ❑ No

25. Do you have any condition limiting the motion of your muscles, joints, or any part of the body that could be aggravated by exercise? ❏ Yes ❏ No
26. Has a physician ever advised you not to exercise? ❏ Yes ❏ No
27. Do you have any suspicion that exercise might be harmful to you? ❏ Yes ❏ No

Answers

If you answered yes to any of these questions, you may need to have an evaluation before exercising, to avoid increasing your risk of heart attack or physical injury.

Safety

Before you begin any fitness program, do the following:

1. Ask your doctor if you can do moderate aerobic exercise.
2. Begin your exercise session with a warm-up and end it with a cooldown.
3. Increase by adding 1 minute to your first day's exercise. Add 30 seconds on each succeeding day. This may be slow, but it helps your body adjust to exercise.
4. Do not overdo it. Never exercise so hard that you cannot carry on a conversation. Never exercise so hard that your heart rate goes over 80% of the maximum for your age (see Target Heart Rate, page 116).
5. Try to avoid exercise that strains your muscles. Muscles that are worked in a new way may be stiff or sore for a day or two. This should go away pretty quickly as your body adjusts to the change. Any pain in a muscle or joint that lasts more than a few days should be evaluated by your health-care provider.

You should always consult a doctor or physical therapist about how or whether to exercise with specific injuries.

Shoes

If you are interested in exercise like walking or climbing stairs, you need comfortable shoes. Your shoes should:

- be flat
- be wide in the front to allow your toes to spread
- have good arch support
- have a rubber sole
- tie instead of slip on or buckle

Feet tend to swell during exercise. Some people wear athletic shoes during their commute to and from work. This helps them make physical activity part of their day. You can carry or keep a pair of dressier shoes at work and walk or climb your way to a new you!

Feet and Diabetes

If you have diabetes, it is especially important to take care of your feet. People who have diabetes may have problems with circulation or lose feeling in their legs and feet. They can quickly develop infections that can lead to serious complications.

It is important to always check your feet thoroughly for sores and bruises after physical activity. If you find a blister, bruise, or cut, bring it to your doctor's attention before it becomes serious. Never perform any activity in high heels or tight shoes. You should also clean and massage your feet often in warm water with products that do not contain perfume or alcohol. Do not put lotion between your toes. Change your socks regularly and always wear shoes (even when you are indoors). Be good to your feet and they will be good to you!

CHAPTER **FOURTEEN**

Exercise Planning

Physical Fitness: Not All or Nothing

Making exercise a permanent part of your life probably requires you to change. Exercise is not something you just do. You need time, energy, and realistic goals.

> *Change is not all or nothing, and it does not happen at one point in time.*

If you view change as having to be all or nothing, you can fall back into old habits and have difficulty starting again. You may blame yourself for being weak-willed. Everyone falls off the wagon now and then. If you recognize this, you will not be so hard on yourself if it happens.

Health clubs count on people relapsing to make money. They recruit more members than they expect to hold. If every health club member came to the club 3 to 6 days a week, it would be so crowded, no one could work out. Health clubs know that most people will join, work out for a few days or a few months, and then stop.

Every problem you confront as you begin is an opportunity to learn—not a sign of failure. Using this perspective has revolutionized treatment for people with addictions. In a way, a sedentary life is an addiction. It is easier to continue not moving. Break the cycle! Start with a walk through the park or around your neighborhood. Decide that today is *your* day to put the past behind you.

Pros and Cons About Physical Activity

Before you can change your lifestyle, you must consider the pros and cons of physical activity. Pros might include helping you lose weight, giving you energy, and feeling in shape. Cons might include time, expense, and effort.

List the pros and cons of participating in physical activity.

Pros	Cons
1. _____	1. _____
2. _____	2. _____
3. _____	3. _____

Stages of Change

There are different stages of change, and each has a series of techniques you can follow. Envision yourself on a journey where each step guides you to the next step. Change is always possible. It begins with you.

The stages of change are not linear but cyclical. Even people with "great bodies" admit that they go through periods without exercise. There are periods, like the beginning of the year, when people are motivated to change, and there are periods, like Thanksgiving, when most of us do not even consider exercising.

Worksheet 14A: Stages of Change

See what stage you are in now. Don't worry! The stage you are in changes all the time. You may do this worksheet again in a week and be in a different stage. There are techniques for each stage that enable you to move on; so wherever you are, you can progress. Find out where you are now. Place a check mark in the box that best describes how you feel.

1. I don't want to exercise.

2. I have thought about exercising, but I haven't actually tried it yet.

3. I have thought about exercising and plan to try in the next month.

4. I have actually begun some type of regular exercise.

5. I work out regularly, but sometimes I don't.

Scoring

Each of the questions above corresponds to the same number below. These are the stages of change.

1. Not ready to exercise

2. Thinking about exercise

3. Getting ready to be physically active

4. Starting exercise

5. Keeping on

Stage 1: Not Ready to Exercise

If you are in this stage, you are not even considering change. You may be trying to deny your current health status or may not be willing to see things in a different way. From time to time, you may experience pressure from others to change. Two change processes seem to work well at this stage, *gathering information* and *ranting and whining*.

Gathering Information

You need to gather more information about yourself, your feelings, and exercise. You can gather information by watching television or movies about sports, reading about exercise, or talking to people who exercise regularly.

Do you think you can motivate yourself to gather information about exercise? If your answer is still no, you are probably not ready to commit to a weight-management program. If your answer is yes, list three ways you can gather information about exercise.

1. _____

2. _____

3. _____

Ranting and Whining

Ranting and whining means expressing your feelings in a way that will gradually change your behavior. When you rant and whine about a situation, you are not satisfied with, you become more aware of what is troubling you. Although ranting and whining may not lead directly to change, it can help you start the process. Your resistance to exercise may be due to your belief that you can't do it, your weight, or disease. Talking and even complaining can increase your awareness of your feelings toward exercise and help you decide what, if any, fitness goals you will set.

Sally's Story

Sally, a woman in her sixties, has rheumatoid arthritis. She complains about it and dramatizes it. Sally's complaints about how hard it is to open jars and move around can be beneficial if they help her understand her problem. Sally's behavior may appear to make the situation worse because she seems to be wallowing in self-pity. But when she has grieved for what she has lost, she can move on to see what she can do about it. By using her feelings, Sally realizes that exercise can make her stronger and more flexible and offset the limitations that the arthritis is putting on her.

If you believe ranting and whining will be helpful to you, list ranting and whining statements below.

1. _____

_____

2. _____

_____

3. _____

_____

Some of you may consider these actions meaningless. Before you form opinions, try them. They may be more enlightening than you realize. If they don't do anything for you, read about the next stages and think about ways you can motivate yourself to reach these stages of change.

Stage 2: Thinking About Exercise

In this stage, you consider the pros and cons of starting a physical fitness plan but are not yet active.

Beginning to think about exercise requires answering a few questions.

- How can I fit physical activity into my lifestyle?
- What forms of physical activity are most appealing to me?
- Do I own a comfortable pair of sneakers or walking shoes?

You will also take a more in-depth look at your perceptions of exercise, your values regarding physical activity, your role models, and ways to reinvent yourself and imagine yourself being more physically active.

Defining Your Values

Is exercise valuable to you? Do you feel it is good, bad, fun, or dreary? Why? Use the following lines to write down your positive and negative feelings about exercise.

Positive Feelings

1. _____

_____

2. _____

_____

3. _____

_____

Negative Feelings

1. _____

_____

2. _____

_____

3. _____

_____

Look at your list. Ask yourself where these feelings come from. How do negative feelings keep you from your goals? How do positive feelings motivate you? Does this help you see how you feel about exercise? Does this help you see how you can approach exercise in a way you haven't before?

Role Models

Role models are a way of gathering information. Look for role models among your friends and acquaintances. Also look for role models while watching sports on television, seeing a martial arts movie, or going to a high school or college sporting event. Choose an activity that you think you might enjoy and can do. Find out more about a person or team that does this activity.

Once you open yourself to the possibilities, there are many physical activities that you can watch. Use your role model to inspire you and motivate you to do these things yourself.

Reinventing Yourself

When you reinvent yourself, you look at yourself in a different way. Have you ever played air guitar, pretending to be a rock musician? This kind of fantasy allows you to try out different roles for yourself. We often do this as children and up through the twenties but stop when we get older. Try imagining yourself as an athlete, a dancer, or someone who is really in shape.

Think about yourself and ways to be more physically active. How would you reinvent yourself? List three new roles for the reinvented you. Be creative. Don't hold back!

1. _____

   _____

2. _____

   _____

3. _____

   _____

Imagery

Imagery involves picturing yourself as more flexible, thinner, or closer to the results you want from your exercise plan. When you close your eyes, you can imagine yourself moving as you would like to move, looking the way you would like to look, and feeling the way you would like to feel. Watch it all in the theater of your mind. When you have captured the image, stop, whether it takes you 5 seconds or 10 minutes. Repeat this exercise two or three times a day. It will help you see yourself in a new way.

Imagery is a way to rehearse the action so that, when you try later, it will be easier. Right now picture yourself at your ideal weight. See yourself doing things that your extra weight prevents you from doing now. The same process works with any physical goal. Picture yourself and the image will motivate you and help you reach your goal. Research shows that people who can imagine themselves going shopping for clothes in a small size are more likely to lose weight to reach that size.

Sit down, lean back, close your eyes, and take a few minutes to imagine yourself doing sports, dancing, or something you have always wanted to do. When you finish, write how you feel.

_____

_____

_____

_____

_____

_____

_____

_____

_____

_____

Have Fun

Another technique to help you stick to a physical activity program is to have fun. Explore activities you enjoy. Try playing a game of tennis or throwing a frisbee with friends.

Stage 3: Getting Ready to Exercise

In this stage, your intentions and behavior gear you up to begin. You may plan to begin next month. You may have taken some unsuccessful action in the past year. You may even be making some small attempts to exercise now.

Examining your feelings, reviewing your pros and cons, and sharing your feelings with others can motivate you to exercise. Let others know you are ready to change!

Making Your Debut

Making your debut means you make a formal statement that the rest of your life will be different from your past. Tell others your plans to become physically active. Get support from family and friends to help keep you motivated. Buy a pair of athletic shoes, a special outfit, or a piece of equipment. Give yourself concrete proof that exercise is important to you.

Matt's Story

Matt was 45 years old and 80 pounds overweight. He had been meaning to exercise for years. He had always liked the idea of jogging, but his knees were very weak. He made a decision to do something. Now, his neighbors see him out walking every morning. He talks about it with his friends, taking care not to bore them. He takes pride in doing this for himself. He has changed the way he sees himself. Matt has made his debut as an exerciser.

Increasing Your Belief in Your Abilities

How you think about your ability to do physical activity can have a major impact on the success of your physical activity program.

What are you saying to yourself about exercise? (I think I can. Maybe. I think I can't.) Whatever level of confidence you have in your ability to change, try being more optimistic. If you are saying I think I can, try saying I know I can. If you are saying, maybe I can, try saying, I think I can. If you are saying, I cannot, try saying, maybe I can or at least I'll try.

What do you say to yourself about exercise?

_____

_____

_____

_____

_____

_____

_____

How could you change what you say to show new confidence in yourself?

_____

_____

_____

_____

_____

_____

_____

Belief in yourself can make or break your motivation. There is often a clash between your dedication to yourself and the expectations of your spouse, partner, family, or friends. They may want you to do more or less than you want to do. They mean well. You can direct this area of your life without separating yourself from these people.

Stage 4: Starting to Exercise

In the fourth stage, you choose an exercise or activity and start doing it. You officially change your behavior to reach your fitness goals. Starting requires a commitment of time and energy.

This is the riskiest stage of change. Many people overdo it. When they hurt or exhaust themselves, they become discouraged and do not want to continue the program. If you have started exercising, you may think you are home free. But true change requires developing skills to keep you from falling back on old habits and being willing to cope with problems as they arise.

Organize your day so that you are prompted to move. Wipe the dust and cobwebs off your exercise equipment. Find your athletic shoes. If you join a gym, make sure it is on the way to work or close enough to visit on your lunch hour or right after work. Don't pick a place that is hard to get to.

Rewards can be especially helpful at the starting stage. Promise yourself a little treat if you follow your fitness plan for a certain amount of time. If your goal is to lose weight, too, your reward probably should not be food, but it could be calling a friend you have not talked to in a while, going to a movie or play, or buying some new clothes.

Stage 5: Keeping On

When you are in the fifth stage, you are successfully overcoming new obstacles that interfere with your fitness plan without losing the gains you have made. It is easy to start exercising, but the exercise equipment stored in closets and the unused gym memberships attest to the difficulty of staying with it. The techniques used to stick with a fitness program are the same techniques you have used to stick with anything else. The tricks that work for you may be different from the ones that work for others. But by talking to others you may learn what works for them and what pitfalls to avoid.

One Couple's Story

Since Chris and Karen began their relationship 6 years ago, Chris steadily put on weight. The extra weight made Chris less physically attractive to Karen. At the same time, she was afraid that if Chris got into shape, he might become more attractive to other woman, and she might lose him.

Finally, Karen told Chris she was concerned about the weight he had put on. She was worried about what it was doing to his health and to their relationship. Chris did not want to lose Karen. More important, he had not been feeling good about himself and knew that losing weight and exercising would improve his self-image as well as his health. He fixed up his old bike and began riding it on weekends. In addition, Chris and Karen began an exercise program together, and their health and relationship improved.

A Quick Review of the Stages of Change

Let's review the stages of change and the techniques that work well at each stage.

Stage	Characteristics	How to deal with this stage
Not ready to exercise	Complaining about how difficult exercise is. Dramatizing how much you hate it.	Gather information about exercise. Rant and whine about exercise. Complain about it! Decide what is most important to you about exercise.
Thinking about exercise	Considering the pros and cons of beginning a fitness plan.	Find positive role models, and motivate yourself. Reinvent yourself. Imagine the person you want to be. Imagine yourself at the weight you want to be. Have fun. Begin doing something physical.

Stage	Characteristics	How to deal with this stage
Getting ready to exercise	Planning ahead and making gradual changes. Beginning to follow your plan and identifying potential problems that could cause you to slip up.	Tell others about the changes you have made. Take pride in yourself. Increase your belief in your abilities, and dedicate your life to this change. Decide what is most important to you about exercise. Make a resolution to change, and believe in your ability to change.
Starting to exercise	Following a regular plan to reach your fitness goals.	Try not to overdo it. Continue with the program. Reward yourself for your accomplishments by calling friends, buying new clothes, or going to a movie.
Keeping on	Overcoming the initial obstacles. Establishing a consistent plan.	Continue with the program no matter what. Take the opportunity to gain insight into problems that may keep you from achieving your fitness goals. Appreciate and maintain your relationships with people who have been supportive.

GO FOR IT NOW! GET UP AND MOVE!

CHAPTER FIFTEEN

In this chapter, you learn
- how to use "working out"
- how to use "working in"
- about taking it one day at a time
- what to do if you miss a session of physical activity

Selecting a Physical Activity Plan

Working Out vs. Working In: Which Is Right for You?

There are two approaches to physical activity:

- Working out: you spend some time each day or week at a specific activity.
- Working in: you take the stairs and park far from your destination so that you walk more.

Whichever approach you choose, remember to always warm up for about 5 minutes. Some people choose to warm up by performing the chosen activity at a very slow rate. At the end of your activity, do not forget to cool down and keep moving slowly for 5 minutes. When you're more fit, you may want to add stretching and weights to your program as well.

Working Out

When you choose working out, you select a set time in your schedule so you are active regularly, a certain number of times per week. Having committed to your schedule, you can design your program to target your specific goals.

It is important to realize that exercise actually gives you more energy for the other things in your life. You will be less stressed, less frazzled, more able to concentrate, and better able to sleep. You learn more about working out in chapter 16.

Working In

If a block of time is scarce, consider working in activities such as walking or climbing stairs as part of your daily life. Working in does not require spending money on equipment.

Here are some ways you can work activity into your life.

Climbing Stairs

Climbing stairs is an aerobic exercise that strengthens the muscles in the legs and buttocks and builds cardiovascular endurance (heart and lungs). The trick to climbing stairs is to check your heart rate, keep it in the range you want, and keep track of how many minutes you spend at it each day.

Walking

Walking is the best possible exercise. The human body was designed for it, and there are lots of places to do it. It requires no special equipment or training except for comfortable shoes. Walking outside when the weather is fair can be lovely, but nature is not always cooperative. In bad weather, shopping malls are an alternative. Some malls encourage walkers and even have formal mall walkers clubs that meet an hour or so before the mall opens.

If you live in a city, there are plenty of opportunities to walk. If you take public transportation, get off one train stop or several bus stops early and walk to your destination. Keep track of the time so you know how long you have walked. A walk can help reorganize your thoughts, provide a fresh insight, or give you a different perspective.

While you are health walking, be conscious of your body's movement. Are you standing straight? Are you breathing slowly, rhythmically, and deeply?

Stand tall, be relaxed, and balance your weight equally on your feet. Do not let your head or stomach drop forward or down, or slump into your hips. Like a puppet, feel a string out of the top of your head pulling you gently upright. Look straight ahead. Keep your ribs lifted to allow room to breathe. Your shoulders should be relaxed and low, not up around your ears. Do not let your head bounce or bob. Use your abdominal muscles, not your back muscles, to support your torso. The length of your stride depends on your leg strength and your flexibility. Your stride may lengthen as you walk more, and if you do some gentle stretches or yoga exercises before or after you walk.

Race Walking

Race walking has some important variations. When you race walk, one foot is on the ground at all times, and your weight-bearing leg is straight at the knee when that leg is directly under your body. This causes your hips to sway as your speed increases. The better you follow these directions, the faster you can race walk, and the more you are protected from impact with the ground. You may want to read a book about racewalking or get someone to show you how to do it correctly.

Keep your back straight. If you slump, you will have difficulty breathing and less flexibility. Your whole body should lean forward slightly.

Bend your elbows at a 90-degree angle while you are racewalking. Emphasize the swing behind the body. Keep your arms close to your sides, and do not punch them forward. As you get experience and for a greater aerobic effect, you can carry 1- to 3-pound weights in your hands.

Each arm swings to counterbalance the opposite leg. Your heel should touch the ground first, and you should roll through the middle and outer part of your foot. Push off on your toes. If your shins hurt after a walk, you are not letting your toes drop down after you push off the ground, and your shin muscles cannot rest.

If you straighten your leg as soon as your heel touches the ground, it will be easy to keep straight when your leg is directly under your body. This may seem unnatural at first, but it feels more natural with practice.

Take It One Day at a Time

Increase your exercise gradually so that you are not too tired or in pain. As you become experienced and more fit, you will actually *enjoy* exercise.

You need to follow a plan. Start with 1 minute the first day and add half a minute the second day and each subsequent day. You may feel that you are going too slowly. You are not. Your body needs time to get used to new demands on it. Exercise changes your body. Your heart beats faster, and it pumps more blood. More blood is delivered to the muscles and to your brain. Muscles swell from this. Between exercise sessions, your heart beats more slowly, your blood pressure is lower, but your metabolism is higher than it was before you began exercising. Repetition of specific activities causes muscles to increase in strength. You build muscle and lose fat.

When you push your body beyond its limits it will hurt. Give your muscles a day to heal, especially if you are working with weights. The workouts of the 70s advised people to "go for the burn." In the 80s, it was "no pain, no gain." This is wrong. If you "burn" and find yourself in pain, you are causing tissue damage, and you may need to slow down or discontinue the activity for a while. Adding half a minute per day pushes the body just hard enough without pain or fatigue.

When You Have Missed a Day

It is all right to miss a day. If you do, repeat your last day's exercise schedule. You can miss up to 3 days and not disrupt your progress. After missing 4 or more days, decrease your exercise time by half a minute for each day you missed after the third day.

What happens if you get sick or injured? If you are suffering from a condition that would be made worse by exercise, such as a fever, chest pain, or muscle strain, don't exercise. Otherwise, go slowly at an easy pace. Build up slowly to the workout time and intensity you had established before you stopped. If you are injured, ask your doctor what your limitations are. Do not overexert yourself. You will come back more rapidly than you realize, if you take the time to heal.

CHAPTER **SIXTEEN**

Aerobic Exercise

Regular aerobic exercise improves the function of your heart and lungs, making each heartbeat and breath more efficient. It also increases endurance, makes physical activity easier, and often improves your self-image. Aerobic exercise can help you maintain good health and increase your energy. It is also the best exercise for weight control.

Heart as a Muscle

When the heart is strong, it can pump blood efficiently and provide your body with the oxygenated blood it needs.

A strong heart

- provides necessary oxygen with fewer beats per minute
- pumps more blood to the muscles per beat
- enables your body to remove waste products more efficiently

> **Question:** How can I strengthen my heart?
> **Answer:** Through regular aerobic exercise.

Your Target Heart Rate

The table helps you determine the target range for your heart rate during aerobic exercise. You want to keep your heart rate between 60 and 80% of what you can do. In other words, don't workout as hard as you can. Keep your efforts in the moderate range to avoid injury and to burn fat.

Target Heart Rate by Age

Age	(beats/minute) 60%	(beats/minute) 80%	beats/6 seconds range
20	120	160	12–16
25	117	156	16–16
30	114	152	11–15
35	111	148	11–15
40	108	144	10–14
45	105	140	10–14
50	102	136	10–14
55	99	132	10–13
60	96	128	9–13
65	93	124	9–12
70	90	120	9–12
75	87	116	9–12
80	84	112	8–11
85	81	108	8–10

How to Measure Your Target Heart Rate

The two easiest places to check your pulse are at your **carotid arteries** (located on either side of the adam's apple) and your **radial artery** (¼ inch inside your wrist on the thumb side; press against the bone 1 inch above the wrist joint). To find your pulse, place the tips of your index and middle fingers on one of these arteries. Do not use your thumb. Press gently; you should feel your pulse beating. Do not worry if you cannot find it right away. To count your pulse, look at a watch or a clock with a second hand. Count the number of heartbeats in 6 seconds, then multiply by 10 to get the number of beats in a minute. For example, if you count 8 beats in 6 seconds, your pulse is 80 **(8 beats x 10 = 80 beats per minute).**

> Practice taking your heart rate now.
>
> My heart rate is _____ beats per minute.

How Long Should I Exercise at My Target Heart Rate?

When you are warmed up and are at your target heart rate, exercise for 20 to 30 minutes. You increase the time over a month or two. At the beginning, check often to see what your heart rate is. As you get more experience, you'll usually know when you are in your heart-rate range, but you should check it occasionally to be sure.

Aerobic Training

Did you know that regular aerobic exercise can reduce feelings of sadness, blues, depression, or anxiety? Aerobic exercise gets blood pumping to the brain and body, bringing oxygen, and carrying away waste. Aerobic exercise increases the production of endorphins and other chemicals in the brain that are known to influence mood. The increase in endorphins produced during exercise gives you greater pain tolerance both during exercise and at rest.

The most helpful kind of physical activity for weight reduction is aerobic exercise. Yoga, stretching, and weight training will help you get truly fit but by themselves will not help you lose weight.

Aerobic exercise is something you want to fit into your life. If 10 minutes is all you can do, begin with 10 minutes twice a week. If it is hard to reach these goals, you can change them. Don't give up.

Exercise wisely.

- Build by only ½ minute per day.
- Start counting your exercise time from when your heart rate reaches 60% of your capacity. Never let it get beyond 80% of your capacity.
- Stop exercising if you are breathing so hard that you can barely speak.

Five Phases of an Exercise Session

Phase 1: Warm-Up

The warm-up gets your blood flowing through the muscles to prepare them for more intense use. Your body is like a car on a cold day; the oil in the engine is thick and needs to be warmed up. During the warm-up, changes in the nerves tell the breathing muscles that exercise will shortly begin. The muscles and joints also have a chance to loosen up and prepare for the exertion.

Warm up gradually by walking slowly, doing calisthenics, or, perhaps, light jogging in place. You should not be fatigued by the warm-up, and your heart rate should increase to within 20 beats of your target rate. If your target rate is 110 beats per minute, then the warm-up should bring you to a pulse of about 90.

Phase 2: Stretching

Because no single stretch can include your entire body, stretching should be done for each joint. Start at the neck and work down to the ankles. Neck rotations, shoulder rolls, and arm swings warm up each area before it is stretched. You want to stretch to the point of tension, but not pain. Hold the stretch for 5 to 30 seconds—no more—and do not bounce as you stretch. Release the stretch. Repeat it, reaching a little farther this time. Consult a health or exercise professional about safe and effective stretches to prevent injury.

Phase 3: Aerobic Activity

After warming up and stretching, you are ready for aerobic activity. As you exercise, check your pulse, and compare it to the target heart rate (page 116).

The aerobic exercise you choose should use the large muscle groups (like the buttocks, thighs, and calves) in a repetitive way to increase the amount of oxygen your muscles use and increase your target heart rate. Aerobic exercises include continuous, interval, circuit, or a combination of circuit and interval. Read about each type and decide which is best for you.

Continuous Aerobic Training

Continuous aerobic training involves exercising for a set amount of time without stopping. You need to be in pretty good shape, so the inexperienced athlete should start slowly. Whether you walk, ride a bike, jog, or cross-country ski, you should exercise briskly enough to reach your target heart rate.

Interval Training

Interval training involves different levels of aerobic activity broken up by periods of rest. It improves cardiovascular fitness better than continuous training. In fact, you can perform more work if you take little rests than by working continuously. Interval training is done by either resting completely or by slowing down every few minutes. If you enjoy jogging, you may want to jog intensely, then reduce your activity to a brisk walk. A good ratio for work to rest time is 1:3. For example, walk quickly for 1 minute, then slow your pace for the next 3 minutes. Keep repeating this until you develop a routine. You can substitute other exercise in these intervals to fit your personal fitness goals.

Circuit Training

Circuit training requires some imagination and planning. Exercises are varied and should include both aerobic and weight-training exercises. For example, you can begin your program by walking on a treadmill and then lift some light weights. Next, you can run on the treadmill or jog in place for a few minutes to burn off the excess fat and calories. You can include isometric exercises. These allow muscles to be tensed against other muscles or against immovable objects. Clenching your fists is an isometric exercise.

A good example of a circuit-training workout would be a session of jumping rope, sit-ups, jogging in place, and isometric exercises.

Combination Training

This is a combination of circuit and interval. You alternate between activities and increase and decrease your level of intensity.

Here is an example of combination training.

- Aerobic: walking (2 minutes)
- Intense aerobic: jogging (1 minute)
- Reducing activity: walking (2 minutes)
- Strengthening: shoulder rolls (4 sets of 20, changing directions)
- Strengthening: shoulder rolls (4 sets of 20 with 3- to 5-lb weights)

> When you begin a fitness program, always go at your own pace. Move briskly but it should not hurt.

In time, you will be used to your routine and may want to change it to something more challenging. Variety keeps you interested and works more muscles more ways!

Phase 4: Cooldown

The cooldown repeats the warm-up movements for 5 to 10 minutes to allow the muscles and joints to slowly return to their preexercise condition. After walking briskly around the block, you should not flop on the couch and cool down by watching television. Rather, walk slowly for another 5 minutes. Unlike the warm-up, your goal is to bring your heart rate down from exertion and to relax your body.

Phase 5: S-T-R-E-T-C-H

They say the best thing about exercise is that it feels so good when you stop. It feels even better when you stretch. Repeat the stretches you did after your warm-up, working from head to toe.

There are many benefits to an aerobic program. Breathing is easier, the heart works better, circulation is improved, muscles have more flexibility and strength, and you have a greater sense of well-being.

Aerobic Activities at Home

You can add aerobic activity to your current lifestyle and perform it regularly at home. Exercising at home has several advantages. You do not have to leave your home, you can wear whatever you feel comfortable in, and everything you need is at your fingertips. Exercise equipment can be very costly, but if you want to make the investment, read on.

Stationary Bike

A stationary bike is an excellent way to burn calories. You can add a reading stand to the handle bars or put the bike in front of the television. The front wheel is usually metal and should be heavy to provide a smooth, even ride. The seat should be easily adjustable and comfortable. The pedals should have toe straps or clips to hold your feet in place. The bike should have a way to easily adjust the pedaling resistance. An rpm (revolutions per minute) meter, an odometer (to determine your mileage), and a timer are helpful.

The stationary bike works your legs and strengthens your heart and lungs. Begin slowly, with only 1 minute on the bike and little if any resistance on the pedal. The seat should be adjusted so that your knee is just slightly bent when the pedal is at the bottom of its circle. Your speed should not be greater than 50 to 60 rpms. Add 30 seconds to your exercise time each session. You will get the greatest cardiovascular benefit if you exercise five days a week.

Stationary bikes vary greatly in price, and it pays to shop around. If you are budget conscious, you can find used bikes at consignment shops, yard sales, and Goodwill and Salvation Army stores. Reconditioned ones are often available at bicycle shops.

Cross-Country Skiing Machine

Another popular piece of home equipment is the cross country skiing machine. This is one of the best forms of exercise for the whole body. Both arms and legs are exercised, and, unlike with a stationary bike, you use additional muscles required to stand up and balance. The equipment should be sturdy and have easily adjustable resistance for both arms and legs. You can adjust the machine to exercise only the legs or only the arms.

Ski machines, like stationary bikes, vary greatly in price. Plan to spend several hundred dollars for one.

Motorized Treadmill

With a treadmill, you can walk daily, regardless of the weather. Using a treadmill allows you to monitor your progress and see how many miles you have walked within a certain time. Some treadmills have an adjustable ramp to make your walk more challenging. Motorized treadmills are expensive, ranging in cost from $1000 to $7000 dollars. Nonmotorized treadmills cost less. Try out different models in the store before buying one, and check whether there is a trial period during which you can return the equipment if you do not like it.

Step Aerobics

Step aerobics is a popular way to burn fat and calories. Most fitness centers have special classes and equipment available. If you prefer to work out at home, step platforms are not very expensive. There are many excellent videotapes you can buy or rent to learn step aerobics. When you are doing step aerobics, make sure your knees bend more than 20 degrees, or you will irritate your kneecap. If this happens, you may need to limit the height of the step. If you do not own a step, you can practice with a small stool, boxes, or a staircase.

When you buy videotapes, make sure you choose a video that is right for your fitness level and taught by a certified physical educator.

Dumbbells and Weights

You can greatly improve your strength and muscle mass—no matter what age you are—by lifting weights. This activity also helps prevent bone loss (osteoporosis). Lifting light weights twice a week is an inexpensive, great way to improve your fitness level quickly. And you can do it while you watch TV!

Many stores sell inexpensive wrist and ankle weights, and you can add heavier dumbbells as you get stronger. But you don't have to buy weights. You can use 1-pound cans, or fill plastic bleach bottles with water, or fill bags with sand.

Lift slowly, and lower the weight slowly. Maintain good posture. Breathe. This is the slowest exercise with the most powerful pay off. When the weights you are using get to be too easy to lift, add one pound.

Fitness Centers

Choosing a Fitness Center

Many fitness centers assume that new members will drop out or rarely visit the facility a few months after they join. Try to obtain a trial membership, and don't be pressured to sign up for a year on the first visit. (Some fitness centers may not even be around for a year.)

A fitness center is a popular exercise option, but choose one carefully. Visit several fitness centers before you join. Go during the time of day you plan to exercise. At popular times, is there a long wait for equipment? Is there a track? Is it crowded? Is prescreening done to set up a program based on your fitness level? Ask if an orientation is given for each piece of equipment. Is the staff helpful and qualified? Are they members of exercise associations? Do they encourage warm-up and cooldowns? Is the staff trained in CPR (cardiopulmonary resuscitation)? What are the lockers like? Is there child care? Are the exercise programs right for you?

Step Aerobics Classes

Most fitness centers offer step aerobics classes. Before beginning these classes, ask for assistance. Have an instructor familiarize you with the different exercises in the routine. A good instructor can observe you and teach you how to get the most out of your workout.

The Future

Vary your activities so you don't get bored and you work different parts of your body. You can find all sorts of physical activities to enjoy. These can include calisthenics, stepping exercises, stretching, racquet sports, dancing, jogging, swimming, cycling, exercise classes, rowing, minitrampolines, walking, in-line skating, basketball, volleyball, tai chi, yoga, martial arts, and weight lifting.

It is good to set goals for how often and how much you exercise, but they should be realistic. Getting out of shape did not happen overnight, so getting into shape will not happen overnight either.

Whatever fitness program you create, make sure you have fun! Stay motivated. You can do it, remember that.

On the following worksheet, write a fitness plan you would be willing to follow for the next few weeks. Next to each day, put the activity you will do and the amount of time you will spend doing it.

Worksheet 16A: My Fitness Plan

Day	Activity	Time Spent on the Activity
Sunday		
Monday		
Tuesday		
Wednesday		
Thursday		
Friday		
Saturday		

Section Four

EMOTIONS &
ROADBLOCKS

CHAPTER **SEVENTEEN**

Feeling Positive About Your Plan

Setting realistic goals is an important part of losing weight. People like immediate satisfaction and want to see that they have lost weight. However, focusing on the scale rather than on a healthy lifestyle can set you up to fail. If you do not lose weight immediately, you may become frustrated and give up. People are most successful if they plan small goals and move on gradually as they master each one.

In the past, you probably set goals for yourself that were too difficult.

Why Setting Realistic Goals Is Important

Unrealistic goals are one of the most common reasons people fail to lose weight.

Unrealistic Goals
- Expecting yourself to follow a very low calorie diet for an extended period.
- Thinking that you will see a noticeable weight loss when you get on the scale each week.
- Believing you can give up one of your favorite foods for the rest of your life. Depriving yourself will only lead to strong cravings, and you will eat even more.
- Becoming so enthusiastic about starting an exercise program that you set goals you cannot meet. Do not start by planning to work out every day and run a marathon.

In the past, when you attempted to lose weight, certain methods and changes worked and others didn't. Think about previous goals that were too difficult to follow. Don't be like Discouraged Debbie.

Discouraged Debbie

Debbie was recently diagnosed with diabetes and is taking medication. She made the following list of goals for herself.

1. I will never eat junk food.

2. I will run five miles a day.

3. I will lose 20 lbs in the next three weeks.

4. I will follow a very strict meal plan of fruits and vegetables.

Within four days, Debbie was craving every food. Her legs were sore from the rigorous activity. She began to feel extremely fatigued, irritable, and confused. After a visit with her doctor, she learned she had been hypoglycemic. She never thought her strict plan would have such an impact on her body. She had not lost weight, she did not have control of her diabetes, and her meal plan was too hard to follow. She wanted to give up.

If Debbie's goals had been reasonable and her changes gradual, she would not have become so discouraged.

Worksheet 17A: Your Unreasonable Goals

List some goals you made in the past that you couldn't reach.

1. _____

_____

2. _____

_____

3. _____

_____

4. _____

_____

Think about why these goals were so difficult. Perhaps they were unreasonable. Maybe now, in this life phase, they are attainable. You need to think about small, reasonable steps to take. You can always add to these, but begin with something you can accomplish! This will build up your confidence and help you truly change your lifestyle.

On paper, this may sound easy,
but how do you go about actually setting realistic goals and following them?

How to Set Realistic Goals

It is important to personalize each goal. Don't just copy someone else. Think about the type of person you are and realize what works for you. Break down each of your goals into the following three steps.

1. Define the problem.
2. Turn the problem into a positive statement.
3. Change the problem into a realistic goal.

Munching Matthew's story will help you understand how to do this for yourself.

Munching Matthew

Define the Problem
Matthew knows that his downfall is eating too many chocolate chip cookies. He cannot help himself. Using a food diary helps him identify the patterns that start his overeating. Certain times, places, and situations are particular triggers.

Turn the problem into a positive statement.

Munching Matthew usually tells himself, "I will never eat another cookie!"

But "Managing" Matthew could say to himself, "As long as I monitor what I eat, I can have three cookies each day."

Change the Problem into a Realistic Goal
Matthew now has a realistic goal. He allows himself some of his favorite foods without going overboard. By following a meal plan or watching fat and calories, he has his cake and eats it, too! Changing his eating habits did not mean he had to deprive himself of his favorite food.

How about goals for including physical activity in your lifestyle?

Sluggish Sally

Sally believes she can never find time to exercise. However, Schedule Sally can look carefully at her excuses not to exercise. Sally thinks about a reasonable plan. She decides to try to walk for 15 to 30 minutes after dinner at least 3 days a week, unless it's raining outside.

> *Remember: Be positive, not negative!*
>
> **Negative:** There's no way I can find time to exercise!
>
> **Positive:** If I can find time for watching TV, I can find time to walk. I am going to walk for 30 minutes after dinner 3 days a week, unless the weather is dreadful. At those times, I'll do stretches and lift some light weights while I watch TV.

Don't make vague statements such as, "I'm going to exercise." Pinpoint the behavior you want, and make a clear statement with the details of what you're going to do.

1. TIMING: When this action will take place.
2. FREQUENCY: How often this action will take place.
3. CIRCUMSTANCES: The situations that will affect this action.

Let's take another look. "I am going to walk for thirty minutes after dinner (TIMING) at least three days a week (FREQUENCY), unless it is raining outside (CIRCUMSTANCES)."

Set realistic goals for yourself. This workbook only serves as a guide to encourage you to use your time and effort in a positive way. You have to make the choice. Take a look at some negative statements that people often make when they are trying to lose weight. Then look at the positive, action-oriented goals that you can develop.

1. *Negative*—I will never touch another cookie as long as I live.
   Positive—It is possible to budget cookies into my weekly plan. If I am careful about counting calories and fat grams, I can include cookies in my meal plan.

2. *Negative*—When I am on the run, it is impossible to eat sensibly.
   Positive—It is possible to plan my meal ahead of time and bring food with me. This way, I am taking charge of my eating and not leaving it to chance that I will find something healthy.

3. *Negative*—My family does not like to eat healthy meals. They complain that these foods have no taste.
   Positive—I will learn how to cook and prepare tasty foods in a healthy way.

Remember, change is an ongoing process. Believe in yourself and you will go far on the road to a healthy lifestyle.

Worksheet 17B: Overcoming Obstacles

Now it is your turn to think of some realistic goals.

Think about your list of unrealistic goals.

Write these or others in the first column, and then write the positive statement that is a reasonable goal.

Remember, your statements should include *timing*, *frequency*, and *circumstances*.

What Didn't Work	What Will Work
1. _____	1. _____
2. _____	2. _____
3. _____	3. _____
4. _____	4. _____
5. _____	5. _____

Changing Your Lifestyle

You decided that you want to change your lifestyle to include eating well and physical activity. Deciding to make a change usually means dropping a bad habit or introducing a good one. But it is not that simple. Changing our behavior requires us to make a series of decisions.

Building Confidence

Are you confident that you can lose weight? Are you confident that you can avoid overeating in every situation? How do you feel about exercising? Are you confident that you can begin a fitness program and stick with it?

Your level of confidence not only determines how well you do something, it is also a pointer to what you might try to do. You are more likely to try something when you think you will succeed than when you believe you will fail.

On the other hand, you may know you can do something but may not think it is worth doing. When considering a change, three questions come to mind:

1. Is it worth doing?
2. Will I try it?
3. Can I do it?

These are the questions to answer when you are thinking about exercising and adopting better eating habits. To answer the first question, collect information on the subject, and decide whether the benefits outweigh the inconvenience. You have been given a lot of information about the benefits of physical activity and eating healthfully to maintain your ideal weight.

Hopefully, you will decide these changes are worth making, but what if you have tried and failed before? Your answer may be that you will not try because you do not think you can do it. You are basing your answer on your previous experiences, which have been discouraging. *This time it can be different!*

It is important to look at your past and think about each time you have tried to lose weight. What factors contributed to your success? What factors led you to fail? The following set of questions help you think about and learn from your previous attempts to lose weight.

Worksheet 18A: Previous Attempts to Lose Weight

1. Recall a time in your past that you successfully lost weight. When did this happen? (month/year) _____

   If there is more than one time, answer the following questions for each time.

2. Where were you when this happened? _____

   Were you doing this alone or did you diet with a partner? _____

   What was happening at this time of your life? _____

   _____

   _____

3. Can you recall how you felt at that time? Did any particular feelings about trying to lose weight stand out? How was your mood during this successful attempt at weight loss? _____

   _____

   _____

4. What was the outcome of your success? How did you feel about it and yourself? How did others treat you and react to your success? _____

   _____

   _____

---

5. What helped you to be successful? How did you eat or exercise? How did you deal with temptations and urges? _____

_____

_____

6. Think about a time you attempted to lose weight and were not successful. (Either you did not lose weight or you gained weight.) List the approximate time in your life (month/year). Why did the attempt fail? _____

_____

_____

7. Think about what was going on around you. Were you alone or with other people? What were you doing at the time? _____

_____

_____

8. What was going on inside you? What kind of feelings prevented you from reaching your goals? _____

_____

_____

9. Did something significant end your attempt to lose weight? What happened? _____

_____

_____

10. How did you feel about yourself? How did others react toward you?

_____

_____

_____

_____

_____

Think about your answers. Do you notice a pattern? Do you believe there was a difference in your approach to weight loss between the times you succeeded and the times you failed? Take a moment to reflect, and write down any patterns you notice.

_____

_____

_____

_____

_____

_____

_____

_____

_____

Behavior Chains

Behavior chains are a series of steps a person goes through to set himself or herself up for a certain behavior, such as eating. In chapter 4, we discussed the ABCs of Eating and how knowing the ABCs can prevent you from overeating. Understanding your antecedents (or the triggers), your behavior (overeating,) and consequences (how you feel after you overeat) can help you break the habits that keep you from success.

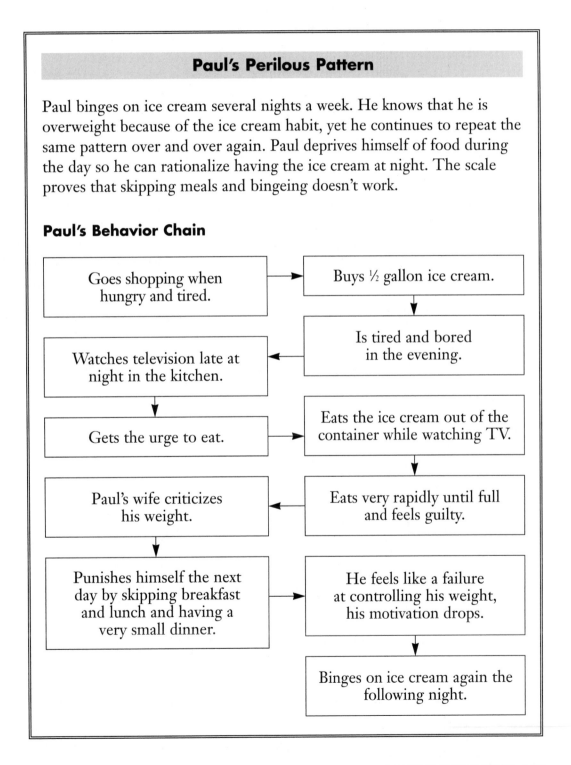

Paul's Perilous Pattern

Paul binges on ice cream several nights a week. He knows that he is overweight because of the ice cream habit, yet he continues to repeat the same pattern over and over again. Paul deprives himself of food during the day so he can rationalize having the ice cream at night. The scale proves that skipping meals and bingeing doesn't work.

Paul's Behavior Chain

Goes shopping when hungry and tired. → Buys ½ gallon ice cream.

Is tired and bored in the evening.

Watches television late at night in the kitchen.

Gets the urge to eat. → Eats the ice cream out of the container while watching TV.

Paul's wife criticizes his weight. ← Eats very rapidly until full and feels guilty.

Punishes himself the next day by skipping breakfast and lunch and having a very small dinner. → He feels like a failure at controlling his weight, his motivation drops.

Binges on ice cream again the following night.

A common mistake people make is expecting to show perfect willpower at the *end* of the chain. You can see from Paul's behavior chain that control becomes more and more difficult as the pattern progresses. The weakest link in Paul's chain, the easiest place for him to break the pattern, is not to buy the ice cream. Recognizing the circumstances that place him at risk for bingeing would give Paul more options for changing things. Changing behavior even at the end of the chain would also help. Going out to an ice cream parlor and buying one scoop of ice cream would fulfill his urge with far fewer calories than the binge at home.

Here are some techniques Paul can use for positive change.

Behavior	Techniques for Change
Buys ½ gallon of ice cream.	1. Shop from a list. 2. Take only enough money to buy the foods on the list. 3. Shop with diet partner, or ask spouse to do shopping. 4. Shop only on a full stomach. 5. Buy a low-calorie pudding that requires preparation instead of buying ice cream. 6. Substitute a nonfood reward as a treat instead of buying the ice cream. 7. If craving for ice cream persists, buy 1 scoop from an ice cream parlor instead of ½ gallon from the grocery store.
Tired and bored in the evening.	1. Get more exercise. 2. Get more sleep.
Watches TV late at night in the kitchen. Gets the urge to eat.	1. List alternatives to eating. 2. Get out of the kitchen. 3. Do not keep TV in the kitchen. 4. Wait 5 minutes, urge may pass. 5. Separate hunger from craving.
Eats very rapidly until full.	1. Put utensil down between bites. 2. Wait 20 minutes before taking second helping.

Behavior	Techniques for Change
Feels guilty.	1. Analyze what went wrong.
Punishes himself the next day by skipping breakfast and lunch and having a very small dinner.	1. Set more realistic goals. 2. Eat three meals during the day so that control will be better at night.
Wife criticizes his weight. Feels like a failure, and motivation decreases.	1. Read workbook for ideas. 2. Check emotions and attitudes.
Binges on ice cream again the following night.	1. Look at behavior chain. Plan techniques to break the chain.

Worksheet 18B: Analyzing Your Own Behavior Chain

Learning to recognize your behavior chains is probably the most important lesson you can learn from this program. Early recognition of the chain in a high-risk situation that leads to overeating gives you more options for change. Use your food diary, or think back to what your old eating habits were, and write out an unhealthy behavior chain. Below, write techniques to use to break each link of that chain.

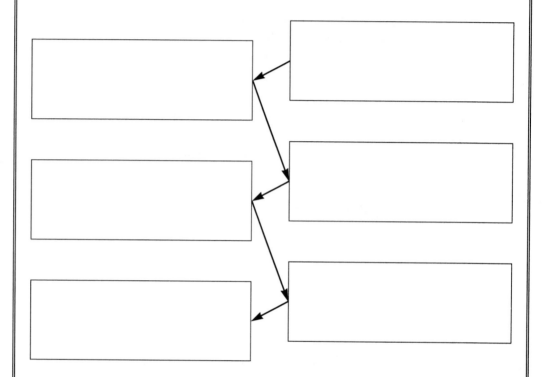

Behavior	Technique for Change

CHAPTER NINETEEN

Dealing With Lapse and Relapse

In the past, you probably tried to lose weight, only to regain it eventually. It is possible to lose a few pounds, but it's not easy to maintain that weight loss. Here we concentrate on coping with situations that trigger overeating or that keep you from exercising.

Lapse vs. Relapse

There is a difference between slipping (a lapse) and losing complete control of your weight-management program (relapsing). When you relapse, you fall back into all of your old ways of behaving. Everyone slips, but it is important to understand the reasons *you* slip so you won't relapse. A relapse is linked to how strongly you believe in your ability to do something. Anytime you try to change behavior, you will only succeed if you believe you can change. Your level of self-confidence may depend on the situation. You may be unsure of yourself in certain situations, or you may be afraid to try new ones. You can probably recall times when you had great faith in your ability in a special situation, often because you had practiced beforehand and succeeded in doing it. It is important to identify the situations that test your self-confidence.

Identifying High-Risk Situations

Becoming aware of your weaknesses is important. When you look at your history of weight loss, you can identify high-risk situations that caused problems. You find situations in which you overate or stopped following your fitness program. Now, when you slip, stop, analyze why you lapsed, and decide what to do differently next time. Analyzing a slip gives you more control over your eating behavior.

Possible high-risk situations

- When you feel negative emotions, such as frustration, anger, and depression
- When you do not feel well
- Celebrations or times when you believe you deserve a treat
- When you cannot pass up a treat or feel pressure from others

The more high-risk situations you can identify, the better you can cope with them. When you can cope, you gain self-confidence. And self-confidence helps you succeed.

Worksheet 19A: Problem Areas

Check the areas that apply to your high-risk situations to help you pinpoint possible problems.

1. ❏ Alone, lonely

2. ❏ Argument with spouse/family

3. ❏ Rejected, depressed

4. ❏ Anxious, tense, nervous

5. ❏ Guilty

6. ❏ Ashamed, embarrassed

7. ❏ Bored

8. ❏ Angry

9. ❏ Stressed about work demands

10. ❏ Frustration

11. ❏ Tension with boss or co-workers

12. ❏ While watching TV

13. ❏ Before going out, in the evening

14. ❏ Procrastination

15. ❏ While talking on the phone

16. ❏ During weekends

17. ❏ Travel for work or vacation

18. ❏ At the movies, circus, sports events

19. ❏ Celebrations (parties, holidays)

20. ❏ While preparing meals/cooking

21. ❏ In a restaurant, cafeteria (buffet)

22. ❏ Bedtime treat/midnight snack

23. ❏ Under pressure to "clean" my plate/not to throw away food

Answers

Look at your answers. They can be divided into three main problem areas. Which one best applies to you?

Negative Feelings

Are most of your checks in statements 1–11? This means that you have a tendency to overeat when you are experiencing a feeling that is uncomfortable for you. Eating probably makes you feel better in the short run, but it has negative consequences in the long run. Not only will you be more likely to gain weight, but you are not learning to manage your emotions appropriately.

Leisure and Unstructured Time

Did most of your checks fall in statements 12–19? You may have difficulty eating well in situations that are not structured or when you are not consciously thinking about food. You may find yourself staring at the TV and, before you know it, you've eaten a pint of ice cream. You need to be aware that times like these are high-risk situations when you eat unconsciously.

Exposure to Food

If you checked off more in statements 18–23, you are likely to eat more when food is in front of you and readily available. At social events, there is usually a large amount of food, and it's easy to eat a lot without being aware of it. Seeing food or thinking about it triggers you to eat more than is healthy for you. You need to prepare ahead when you know you are going to be around food.

Worksheet 19B: Physical Activity

Not following your fitness plan is also a slip. Think about the times when you did not feel like exercising or had a hard time exercising regularly. The following list includes reasons you may not have felt like moving! Check the ones that apply to you. (Add any others that apply to your situation.)

1. ❏ I don't have enough time.

2. ❏ I'm too tired.

3. ❏ I can't afford it.

4. ❏ The weather is uncomfortable.

5. ❏ My family/friends do not seem to be supportive.

6. ❏ I don't like to wear exercise clothes.

7. _____

8. _____

9. _____

10. _____

Answers

1. No time
There are two types of exercise, a formal exercise program, such as running 3 miles a day, and lifestyle exercise, which is an increase in your daily physical activity. When you can't find time for formal exercise, remember there are things you can do.

- Park the car a distance from your destination and walk.
- Use the stairs when possible, not the elevator or escalator.
- Take dancing lessons, or dance around the house.
- Kill two birds with one stone—do some housecleaning.
- Fitness walk on your lunch hour. Take a friend.

Making exercise a priority in your life is important. It is the secret to success in a weight-loss program. Exercising can actually increase your time. Why? Because your energy level will go up, and you will be more productive. A half-hour walk in the morning to begin your day is better than caffeine to get you up to speed.

2. Tiredness

Exercise increases your energy. You will feel younger and be able to manage your time better. Exercise is an excellent way to combat stress, and stress is often what makes you feel exhausted and unproductive. Exercise also improves sleep and sharpens your thinking.

3. Expense

Do not feel that you must join a gym or health club. Walking is a wonderful way to get exercise. It is simple, pleasant, and one of the most effective forms of physical activity. Start off slowly by walking 10 minutes a day. Increase your time gradually until you walk 30 to 40 minutes, three days a week. Your only expense is a good pair of shoes.

4. Weather

Once you begin exercising, the weather should not stop you. A walk in the rain or snow is a rich experience. Dress appropriately. When it's too hot or too cold, you can work out at home or another convenient location. You might want to buy a workout tape if you have access to a VCR. Or you can check for regularly scheduled exercise shows on television. Videos and TV shows cover all levels of fitness in exercise from aerobics to yoga to weight lifting.

5. Lack of support

Tell your family and friends that you are changing your lifestyle. Ask the important people in your life for support. When they know how important your goals are to you, these people are more likely to encourage you. If you include them, you can all support each other! Exercising with your family is a great way to spend quality time together. Working out with others motivates you to keep on moving.

Aggravated Angelo

Angelo has struggled with his weight for most of his life and often feels he has no control. After he developed diabetes, he found it more difficult to talk with his friends and family about his weight loss goals because they were quick to tell him what he was doing wrong. He understood that they are concerned about his health, he only wished that they would stop saying "Don't eat those donuts! Stay away from that cake!"

Instead of staying aggravated, Angelo discussed his feelings with his family and friends. They agreed not to criticize him. They learned to support him in positive ways. Now, he takes daily walks with his neighbor and helps his wife prepare foods that he enjoys. He is happy that he shared his feelings and appreciates the support he receives from his friends and family.

Coping With Lapse and Relapse

When you are unprepared for a situation, you're more likely to "slip." This lapse feels like a loss of control. But losing control once or twice does not mean you have completely relapsed. The lapse is an opportunity to examine what went wrong and a way to learn for the future. Think about walking along an icy road. You might slip and lose your balance. Instead of falling down, you regain control, walk more slowly, and keep your balance. In walking down the icy road of weight management, the goal is to learn from your slips and prevent a fall.

STOP! What is happening right now?
LOOK! What is going on around me?
LISTEN! How do I feel inside?

Stay calm. Do not waste time or energy feeling guilty. Allow yourself to make mistakes. Examine your feelings, and keep things in perspective. This is one slip. You have not lost complete control over your weight-management program. Expect mistakes, and learn from them. Praise yourself for what you have done correctly. Remember, nobody is perfect.

Rethink your commitment to losing weight. Why did you join this weight-management program? What are your goals? What have you learned and accomplished? For example,

1. I have lost 5 pounds.
2. I have more energy.
3. I am learning to cook exciting and nutritious meals.

Call someone. Just talking to someone who is supportive of you can help. It gets you out of your own mental state and helps you be more objective. If you find that you cannot speak to anyone, write down your feelings on a piece of paper or in a journal. Seeing your feelings on paper enables you to distance yourself and gain a better perspective.

Worksheet 19C: Reviewing the Situation

When you slip do you end up blaming yourself? Think about the situation objectively and what triggered the behavior. What could you have done differently? Write down some ways that you might have prevented the slip. Keep this list handy.

1. _____

2. _____

3. _____

4. _____

5. _____

Remember, slips are normal and you should expect them. The actual slip is not really the problem. The problem occurs if you can't get back on your feet again and continue toward your goals. Make a plan so that slip won't happen again.

I slip when _____

I will avoid this in the future by _____

Obstacles that may come up include _____

I will handle them by _____

Worksheet 19D: Preventing a Lapse

In a high-risk situation, ask yourself these questions:

1. Do I really want to eat this food? ❑ Yes ❑ No ❑ Don't Know

2. How will I feel after I eat this? _____

3. How will I feel if I do not eat this? _____

4. Is eating this worth it? ❑ Yes ❑ No ❑ Don't Know

In the 1st column, list what triggers you to overeat (high-risk situations).
In the 2nd column, list ways to deal with these situations. See the example.

Personal triggers	How can I prevent them?
1. Eating at parties.	1. Eat low-calorie snacks before going out.
2. Munching while watching television	2. Ride the exercise bike while watching TV, or keep my hands busy (knit, pet the dog, etc).

CHAPTER **TWENTY**

Negative Thinking

You may find your weight-management program difficult to follow. Your attitude—your state of mind or feeling—can affect your ability to lose weight. This roadblock can be removed once you understand your attitudes and replace them with positive thinking.

Negative Thinking and Attitude Traps

Self-awareness is a crucial part of losing weight. You need to be aware of inner dialogues or self-talk that result in negative thinking. Negative thinking can lead to problems in your effort to lose weight. You can learn to eject your mental tape and put in a new one.

You have learned about high-risk situations and how they can lead to a lapse. Usually these triggers involve

- negative emotional states
- conflict with others (family, work, or friends)
- social situations (celebrations or parties)

The most powerful of these are the negative emotional states—the bad things you think about yourself. The people you're with or the party situation may call up negative feelings about you. Then you lapse, and you feel guilty, ashamed, and out of control. When you feel this way, you talk yourself into believing the worst about yourself. Confronting this negative self-talk gives you the power to start succeeding with weight loss. You need to believe in yourself and encourage yourself.

Self-destructive Attitudes and Negative Thinking

1. All-or-nothing Thinking

Do you look at things in black-and-white terms? Think of a light switch. It is either on or off, there is no in-between. This type of thinking is rigid. If you say, "I will never eat sweets again!" there is no middle ground. When you give in to that sweet tooth, you tell yourself "I blew it. I might as well eat the whole thing and forget my diet." Feelings of failure lead to overeating. When it comes to eating, never say never! Moderation is the key.

2. Magnification

Do you blow things out of proportion? Do you focus so strongly on your mistakes that you forget your good qualities? This can happen when you eat more than you want and you believe it is the worst thing in the world. Negative emotions can trigger more eating. Pick yourself up. Try again tomorrow. It's not the end of the world.

3. Jumping to Conclusions and Self-fulfilling Prophecies

Do you make negative predictions about the future? "I will never be able to exercise. I will never be able to control my eating." Is this what you want to be true? You cannot tell the future, but you can do certain things today. Have you ever decided that people are reacting negatively to you when the fact is that you are feeling depressed? In trying to predict what others think and feel, we often end up projecting our own negative thoughts and feelings onto them.

4. Should Statements

Do you criticize yourself (or others) with shoulds, oughts, or musts? People who slip often say to themselves, "I shouldn't have done that," and feel guilty. People who feel very guilty relapse more than those who do not. Who makes up those rules? Where did you learn them? Shoulds are only suggestions. You decide what is right for you to do.

5. Discounting the Positive

Do you insist that your accomplishments or good qualities don't count? Acknowledge your successes as you meet your daily goals. Don't overlook your special qualities. When you focus just on the negatives, you take the joy from your life. When you make a mistake, don't label yourself a loser or failure. Making a mistake does not mean that you are that mistake. Say thank you when someone comments on your achievements—don't pretend it's not a big deal.

6. Personalizing

Do you blame yourself for something you are not responsible for? This can happen when you are not being objective, especially when you believe your *feelings* are fact. If you feel bad, then you may think something is your fault. You are reacting to your negative feelings. Review the situation and look at all sides. What part did you play in it? What part did others play? What have you learned?

Negative emotions linked to a small lapse can trigger a full relapse. Let's look at Negative Nancy.

Negative Nancy

Nancy had a tough day at the office and had no time to eat lunch. She came home from work, exhausted and stressed, and went straight to the kitchen. A large bag of potato chips was on the counter. Nancy was starving, and before she knew it, she had eaten the whole bag. At this point, Nancy said to herself, "I should not have done that. I have blown my whole diet. I might as well continue eating, since it doesn't matter anyway. I will never be able to lose weight. I will always be fat."

Problem Solving

To learn from Nancy's lapse, you must understand what happened.

Identify the high-risk situation. Nancy was tired and had not eaten during the day.

Identify the negative self-talk. "I've blown it. I'll never be able to do this."

Identify the negative thinking. "I shouldn't have done that." A should statement leads to self-criticism or punishment.

"I've blown my whole diet." This is all-or-nothing thinking and magnification.

"I might as well continue eating since it doesn't matter anyway." This is dwelling on the negative and discounting the positive. She just made one mistake.

"I will never be able to lose weight. I will always be fat." This is jumping to conclusions and all-or-nothing thinking.

You now have some idea about your negative attitudes and feelings. What you may not realize is that automatic thoughts—the way you speak to yourself—can cause you stress. By changing the way you think, you can control this stress that affects your behavior. Our automatic thoughts are the verbal messages we give ourselves, but they have to come from somewhere. You can change them by examining your core beliefs.

Core Beliefs

Core beliefs are your absolute, deeply ingrained beliefs that you may never have thought about. A core belief could be, "I'm inadequate unless I'm perfect." To change your automatic thoughts, you must identify your core beliefs. Core beliefs lead to assumptions, which trigger automatic thoughts.

Assumptions

Assumptions are if/then statements. For example, If people really get a chance to know me, then they will reject me. Underlying the assumption are your core beliefs that you are not an interesting or likable person. It works like this:

---

core beliefs ➔ assumptions ➔ automatic thoughts

Our beliefs help us make sense of our world but can also create anxiety. You may believe that life is a struggle. You assume that is true, but it is actually something you learned from others. It may not be true. Beliefs create your attitude or feelings. Look at the following statements, and think about whether you believe them.

Worksheet 20A: Core Beliefs

Read the following statements and put a check next to the ones that apply to you.

❏ I need to have love and approval from peers, family, and friends to be worthwhile.

❏ I must not fail or make a mistake. I must be a success.

❏ Life should be easy, and I should not be frustrated. I can achieve happiness through passivity and inaction.

❏ I should always be in control of my emotions. I should be able to control negative feelings, never showing unhappiness or depression.

❏ I should never argue with someone I love.

❏ If I am alone, I will be miserable and not feel worthwhile.

❏ It is horrible when things or people are not as I expect them to be.

❏ All evil and wicked people should be punished.

❏ If someone criticizes me, something is wrong with me.

❏ I must live up to other people's expectations.

❏ I am ugly unless I have a perfect outward appearance.

❏ My worth depends on my achievements, intelligence, status, or attractiveness.

Answers

If you checked 6 or more statements, you seem to view the world as all good or all bad. You are likely to be hard on yourself if you do not reach your weight-loss goal.

If you checked 3–6 statements, you are being too hard on yourself. Your tendency to be rigid may leave you feeling bad when you make mistakes or when things fall below your expectations.

If you checked fewer than 3 statements, you have positive views about life. You are more likely to set realistic goals and not to be discouraged when things do not go as you had planned.

Worksheet 20B: Changing Automatic Thinking

Core beliefs feed automatic thinking. Mistaken core beliefs lead to negative thinking. You've got the wrong idea about who you are and what you can do. Automatic thoughts may affect your behavior without you realizing it. How do you change this? First, it is important to recognize what your automatic thoughts are. Ask yourself these questions about a recent difficult situation.

What was going through my mind—pictures or memories?
Whose voice did I hear inside my head? What was it saying?
What were my feelings?

Answer the following questions to help you identify an automatic thought that isn't helping you. You may want to read the example on page 159 before giving your own answers.

1. Write down a specific situation that creates upsetting emotions for you again and again. This is called the *event*. _____

   _____

   _____

   _____

2. Write down your thoughts about this. These are your worries, judgments, and assumptions about yourself. _____

   _____

   _____

   _____

3. Write down your feelings. What do you feel when you hear these negative statements in your head? What are the emotions that rise from your automatic thoughts? (Use *feeling* words such as *angry, depressed, lonely, frustrated*) _____

   _____

   _____

4. To get rid of critical automatic thoughts and change your feelings, ask yourself the following:

    a.   Is there any real support for this thought? _____

    b.   Do I have evidence that this idea about myself is incorrect? _____

    c.   What is the worst thing that could happen to me? _____

        _____

    d.   What is the best thing that could happen to me? _____

        _____

5. Write down your positive thoughts and feelings that come from facing your ideas about yourself. _____

_____

_____

Example

1. Event: My friend canceled a date for this evening.

2. Negative thinking: He doesn't want to spend time with me because he does not like me. I'm going to be all alone. Nobody likes me. This always happens. I feel empty and worthless.

3. Feelings: Depressed, lonely, sad, scared, hopeless.

4. a. Is there real support for these ideas? No!
   b. Is there evidence that these ideas are false? Although I would have rather gone on a date, being alone can be fun, too. It gives me time for myself. As soon as I get over the disappointment, I will realize that being alone will be peaceful tonight.
   c. Worst thing? I could continue to feel disappointed and not enjoy myself this evening.
   d. Best thing? I will feel more self-reliant and strong. I will realize that it's okay to be alone.

5. Positive thoughts? I'm okay. I'll rent a movie tonight and make a good and healthy dinner. I like some leisure time alone.

An event that originally sparked negative feelings can be seen for what it really is. It does not have to alter your mood drastically. You do not have to react negatively and indulge in food to deal with your negative feelings.

Ways to Restructure Your Thinking

Once you have become aware of automatic thoughts, it's possible to substitute positive ones for the negative ones, as in the example above. The following techniques also help you do this. Each method can help you change your negative thinking.

1. **Identify the Negative Thinking.** Using the checklist of common attitudes and thinking on pages 152–153, write down each negative thought. This will make it easier to think of a positive replacement.

Irrational Isabelle

Isabelle was eating lunch at her work cafeteria when she was joined by some co-workers. Someone had brought in cake and cookies to share with everyone. Before she knew it, Isabelle ended up having more than she meant to have of cookies. Afterward, she felt awful for eating so many cookies. She felt she will never be able to lose weight because she keeps on making mistakes. She decided to forget her whole weight-loss program, because it wasn't worth it anyway.

a. The negative thought: I'm going to give up on my weight-loss efforts because I ate too many cookies.
   Feelings: awful, overwhelmed, and hopeless

b. Common attitude used: All-or-nothing thinking, discounting the positive

c. From the situation you wrote about on page 157, choose a negative thought with accompanying feeling.

   _____ (thought)

   _____ (feeling)

d. Identify what common attitude or thinking you used (all-or-nothing thinking, jumping to conclusions, etc.). _____

   _____

   _____

   _____

e. Now substitute a thought that is more realistic. _____

   _____

   _____

   _____

2. **Examine the Evidence.** Instead of assuming that a negative thought is true, examine the actual evidence for it. Ask yourself, "What evidence supports this thought?" Because we feel terrible, we often believe things are bad without examining the facts.

3. **The Talk-to-Your-Friend Technique.** Talk to yourself the same way you talk to a dear friend who is upset. When a friend makes a mistake, you don't yell at them. You offer support and encouragement. Do the same for yourself. Listen to how you talk to yourself inside your head.

4. **The Goal-Setting Technique.** Do an experiment to test how real your negative thought is. For example, if you believe you always make mistakes and are so stupid, you may not take risks and try to do certain things. Choose a task to test how realistic your thoughts are. You'll see that you can succeed at doing things and that you can learn from your mistakes. Everyone has to make mistakes. It has nothing to do with how smart you are. Create realistic goals and take some chances to overcome the negative thoughts. This will help you put your feelings in perspective.

5. **Thinking in Shades of Gray.** Instead of thinking about your problems in black-or-white terms, view things in shades of gray. Nothing is all right or all wrong. When you have made a mistake that prevents you from following your daily plan, do not say "I've blown it." View it objectively, evaluate the situation, and take the necessary steps to change it.

6. **The Survey Method.** Do a survey to find out whether your thoughts and attitudes are realistic. Ask people who are close to you for a reality check. Explain your thoughts to them and ask for feedback.

7. **No Name Calling.** When you label yourself as inferior or a loser, ask yourself what you mean. Look at what you do, and learn from it. Do not focus on what you think you are.

8. **Watch Your Language.** Substitute calmer, kinder language for should statements and labels. For example, use phrases like "it would be nice" or "it would be preferable" and labels such as *persistent* and *dedicated*.

9. **No Blame.** Instead of blaming yourself for a problem, think about all the factors that may have contributed to it. Be objective. Blame does not solve anything—don't waste your time.

10. **The Cost-Benefit Analysis.** List the advantages and disadvantages of a negative feeling, thought, belief, or behavior. Answer the question, "How does it help me to believe this negative thought, and how does it hurt me?"

List the negative thought. _____

_____

Advantages of believing this	Disadvantages of believing this

11. **Vertical-Arrow Technique.** This technique charts what negative thinking does to you. First, identify the negative thought about a situation that is upsetting you. _____

_____

_____

↓ Draw a downward arrow below it and answer the question, "If this thought were true, why would it upset me? What would it mean to me?"

↓
↓

Write down your second thought. _____

↓

↓ Ask "why would this upset me?" _____

Keep asking this. It will help you see what is behind the negative thinking. Try to see what you are truly afraid of.

- What are the advantages and disadvantages of believing this about yourself?
- What are the *consequences* of believing this?
- Is your core belief realistic?

Be on guard for automatic thoughts, catch them, and question them. You may use any and all of these techniques to change negative thinking. Then, you'll be free to respond to the *event* in new, more satisfying ways.

Coping With Cravings

Cravings can become so powerful, you almost feel as if you are being taken over by another being. You are determined to fight this evil internal monster telling you that you must have that gallon of ice cream. However, the battle is often lost, and you end up overeating. It's important to ask yourself:

1. What are the problem foods that I often eat in high-risk situations, such as at a party, in front of the television, or with friends?
2. How do I react when I feel the urge to overeat?
3. Is there something else I can do?

Cravings

Cravings are not subtle. All of a sudden, your mind seems to lock on to a particular thought—I must have that slice of pizza! You begin to battle with yourself: No, I can't have that pizza. But I must have that pizza. I can't have that pizza. I must have that pizza.

Then, the monster rears up and declares, "I will have that pizza!"

What began as a small swell in the ocean turns into a tidal wave and knocks you down. You need to realize that cravings are feelings that will pass if you give them enough time. The key is to ride out that wave!

Develop Coping Strategies

Obviously, cravings that lead to overeating can interfere with losing weight. There are strategies to help you manage these powerful urges. You can

- limit accessibility—make it more difficult to get those foods
- examine your behavior
- maintain a balanced perspective
- learn the difference between hunger and appetite

Limit Accessibility

You can limit the amount of food you eat by controlling the serving size. Buy only one donut, not a whole box. Eating a small amount and throwing the rest of it away is not a crime. Put foods away when you come home from grocery shopping. Out of sight, out of mind! When you do eat, focus on the taste, texture, and flavor of the food. Eat slowly, breathe between bites. Make eating an enjoyable sensation that you savor, not rush through.

Examine Behavior Patterns

You know the old saying, What you don't know can't hurt you. It's not true. Knowing how you behave helps you see when behavior is helpful and when it can sabotage your weight-loss program. Once you know your particular style of eating and the behavior surrounding it, you can plan for the future. Get to know your patterns. You may need to avoid high-risk situations. If you use food to cope with problems or emotions, find other ways to cope. Examine your cravings to deal with the problem. Look at what Careless Carrie does.

Careless Carrie

Carrie eats a pint of ice cream 3 nights a week. She knows she is overweight and eating this ice cream keeps her from losing weight. Still, she continues this behavior. Carrie will not eat during the day so that she can eat ice cream at night.

Why does Carrie turn to ice cream?

1. She's upset about her weight.

2. She is punishing herself for eating ice cream at night. But depriving herself during the day only leads to greater cravings.

3. She often eats while "spacing out" in front of the television.

How did Carrie break this pattern and become a winner?

1. She planned her meals throughout the day and ate them, so she was not starving at night.

2. She spoke to friends and her spouse about her feelings, and they provided support.

3. She went for short walks in the evening instead of plopping down in front of the television.

4. When she really craved ice cream, she made a smart choice and ate low-fat frozen yogurt instead, very slowly.

You can cope in high-risk situations by

- recording the food you eat in your diary
- asking your friends and family for support
- examining your habits and problem areas
- buying smaller portions of your favorite foods
- planning ahead, making sure you have some good food choices in your cupboards and refrigerator

Maintain a Balanced Perspective

Everyone makes mistakes. That is what makes us human. The trick is not to turn a mistake into a catastrophe. What should you do when you think you have blown it?

NOTHING!

Don't beat yourself up for having an occasional setback. Instead, take a moment to step back and get it in perspective. How important is this moment over the long run?

What can you learn from this situation? "Reframe" what happened so that you can learn from it. Look at it a different way. One meal will not make you gain weight. It's what you do daily that adds up.

Practice delaying your cravings. When the urge hits, remind yourself that the food will always be there. Try to ride it out. During this moment, think about other things you can do instead of giving in to that craving.

Hunger vs. Appetite

It seems simple—eat when you're hungry. Do you know when you're hungry? What is the difference between hunger and appetite? Hunger is your body's natural response to a lack of food. Appetite is a strong desire or craving for food. Hunger is your body talking. Appetite is your mind talking. Because appetite is learned, at times it is confused with hunger.

HUNGER = INSTINCT
APPETITE = DESIRE

(adapted from *Fat Is a Feminist Issue*, by Susie Orbach)

Here are some examples of eating for reasons other than hunger. Some are familiar to you because we've been looking at all the cues that lead you to overeat. Remember the difference between hunger, a gnawing feeling in your stomach, and appetite, eating for taste and sensation from food.

Food Is Social. "I'm very hungry at suppertime, but I like everyone to eat together, because it feels like we are a happy family if we eat together. Mealtimes are significant, not for the food but for the appearance of family closeness."

Mouth Hunger. "I really need to put some food in my mouth; although I don't feel stomach hunger."

Eating Just in Case. "I'm not hungry at the moment, but I might be hungry in a couple of hours. I won't be able to get anything then, so I'd better have some food now."

Deserved Food. "I had a ghastly day. I think I'll cheer myself up with a nice snack."

Guaranteed Pleasure. "Eating goodies is the only way to give myself a real treat. It's the one pleasure I know how to give myself."

Nervous Eating. "I just have to have something. What can I cram into my mouth?"

Celebratory Eating. "I had such a great day, one packet of chips can't hurt me. I deserve a treat."

Eating Out of Boredom. "I'm not in the mood to do anything at the moment. I think I'll fix myself a club sandwich."

Try to eat only when your stomach says it's time.

How Can Exercise Help?

Exercise can help overcome those nasty cravings! Exercise is

- an appetite suppressant
- a way to control stress and stress-induced eating
- a wonderful way to build self-esteem because it increases feelings of well-being
- a way to improve your mental capacity and make you feel vigorous
- an activity that can be enjoyed with others—or alone

Coping With Stress

How can I deal with cravings and cope with stress?

Use the Weekly Stress Inventory on the following pages to identify your main causes of stress. Then come up with ideas for dealing with them. Here are some clues of what to look for.

- Do other people make you anxious?
- Are you always short of time?
- Do short delays in traffic or on the checkout line drive you crazy?
- Are you trying to soar with eagles when you work with turkeys?
- Do you find that you stew over problems with others rather than saying something?
- Are your family members a problem?

Worksheet 21A: Weekly Stress Inventory

Here is a list of stressful events. Read each item carefully. If an event did not happen in the last week, circle the X. If it did happen, show the amount of stress that it caused you by circling a number from 1 to 6 (see scale below). If the event happened 3 or more times during the past week, put a check in the box to the far left.

X—Did not
1—Not stressful
2—Slightly stressful
3—Mildly stressful
4—Moderately stressful
5—Very stressful
6—Extremely stressful

↓ Check if item happened 3 or more times this week

❑ Job or assignment was overdue	X	1	2	3	4	5	6
❑ Was bothered with red tape	X	1	2	3	4	5	6
❑ Argued with a co-worker	X	1	2	3	4	5	6
❑ Customers or clients gave you a hard time	X	1	2	3	4	5	6
❑ Did poorly at a job, task, or chore	X	1	2	3	4	5	6
❑ Hurried to meet a deadline	X	1	2	3	4	5	6
❑ Were interrupted during a job, activity, or thinking	X	1	2	3	4	5	6
❑ Someone spoiled your completed job, task, or chore	X	1	2	3	4	5	6
❑ Did something you were not good at	X	1	2	3	4	5	6
❑ Unable to finish job, task, or chore	X	1	2	3	4	5	6
❑ Unable to finish all plans for the week	X	1	2	3	4	5	6
❑ Were late for work or appointment	X	1	2	3	4	5	6
❑ Were graded or evaluated on your performance	X	1	2	3	4	5	6
❑ Worked late or overtime	X	1	2	3	4	5	6
❑ Not enough money for basics (food, clothing, etc.)	X	1	2	3	4	5	6
❑ Ran out of pocket money	X	1	2	3	4	5	6
❑ Had unexpected bills (traffic fines, etc.)	X	1	2	3	4	5	6
❑ Had problems paying bills	X	1	2	3	4	5	6
❑ Not enough money for fun or recreation (movie, eating out)	X	1	2	3	4	5	6
❑ Had problem obtaining ride or transportation	X	1	2	3	4	5	6

❏ Drove under bad conditions (traffic, weather)	X	1	2	3	4	5	6
❏ Had car trouble	X	1	2	3	4	5	6
❏ Had minor car accident	X	1	2	3	4	5	6
❏ Argued with husband, wife, boyfriend, or girlfriend	X	1	2	3	4	5	6
❏ Child misbehaved	X	1	2	3	4	5	6
❏ Child had school problems	X	1	2	3	4	5	6
❏ Husband, wife, child, or loved one was ill	X	1	2	3	4	5	6
❏ Spouse had problems at work	X	1	2	3	4	5	6
❏ Not enough time for family and friends	X	1	2	3	4	5	6
❏ Had crime in the neighborhood	X	1	2	3	4	5	6
❏ Had household chores (shopping, cooking etc.)	X	1	2	3	4	5	6
❏ Had minor home repairs	X	1	2	3	4	5	6
❏ Had problems with neighbors	X	1	2	3	4	5	6
❏ Ran out of food or personal item	X	1	2	3	4	5	6
❏ Your property was damaged	X	1	2	3	4	5	6
❏ Store did not have something you wanted	X	1	2	3	4	5	6
❏ Had problems with pet	X	1	2	3	4	5	6
❏ Heard a rumor or something bad about you	X	1	2	3	4	5	6
❏ Were told what to do	X	1	2	3	4	5	6
❏ Were lied to, fooled, or tricked	X	1	2	3	4	5	6
❏ Were misunderstood or misquoted	X	1	2	3	4	5	6
❏ Had confrontation with someone of authority (police, boss)	X	1	2	3	4	5	6
❏ Were criticized or verbally attacked	X	1	2	3	4	5	6
❏ Were around unpleasant people (drunk, bigot, rude)	X	1	2	3	4	5	6
❏ Had unexpected guests	X	1	2	3	4	5	6
❏ Did poorly because of others	X	1	2	3	4	5	6
❏ Were forced to socialize	X	1	2	3	4	5	6
❏ Someone broke a promise	X	1	2	3	4	5	6
❏ Someone broke an appointment	X	1	2	3	4	5	6
❏ Competed with someone	X	1	2	3	4	5	6
❏ Argued with a friend	X	1	2	3	4	5	6
❏ Not enough time to socialize	X	1	2	3	4	5	6
❏ Were ignored by others	X	1	2	3	4	5	6
❏ Had someone disagree with you	X	1	2	3	4	5	6
❏ Spoke or performed in public	X	1	2	3	4	5	6
❏ Were interrupted while talking	X	1	2	3	4	5	6
❏ Were stared at	X	1	2	3	4	5	6
❏ Had someone cut in front of you in line	X	1	2	3	4	5	6
❏ Were unable to express self clearly	X	1	2	3	4	5	6

❏ Had unwanted physical contact (crowded)	X	1	2	3	4	5	6
❏ Dealt with rude waiter or salesperson	X	1	2	3	4	5	6
❏ Had no privacy	X	1	2	3	4	5	6
❏ Were excluded or left out	X	1	2	3	4	5	6
❏ Had too many responsibilities	X	1	2	3	4	5	6
❏ Had to make important decision	X	1	2	3	4	5	6
❏ Did not hear from someone you expected to hear from	X	1	2	3	4	5	6
❏ Were disturbed while trying to sleep	X	1	2	3	4	5	6
❏ Forgot something	X	1	2	3	4	5	6
❏ Heard some bad news	X	1	2	3	4	5	6
❏ Were clumsy (spilled or knocked something over)	X	1	2	3	4	5	6
❏ Lost or misplaced something (wallet, keys)	X	1	2	3	4	5	6
❏ Had legal problems	X	1	2	3	4	5	6
❏ Waited longer than you wanted	X	1	2	3	4	5	6
❏ Did something you did not want to do	X	1	2	3	4	5	6
❏ Had to face a feared situation or object	X	1	2	3	4	5	6
❏ Encountered pet peeve (someone failed to knock, etc.)	X	1	2	3	4	5	6
❏ Failed to understand something	X	1	2	3	4	5	6
❏ Had close escape from danger	X	1	2	3	4	5	6
❏ Had minor accident (broke something, tore clothing)	X	1	2	3	4	5	6
❏ Someone borrowed something without asking	X	1	2	3	4	5	6
❏ Had minor injury (stubbed toe, sprained ankle, etc.)	X	1	2	3	4	5	6
❏ Were physically uncomfortable (cold, wet, hungry)	X	1	2	3	4	5	6
❏ Stopped unwanted habit (smoking, overeating, etc.)	X	1	2	3	4	5	6
❏ Were interrupted while relaxing	X	1	2	3	4	5	6
❏ Not enough time for fun or recreation (movie, eating out)	X	1	2	3	4	5	6
❏ Did poorly at sport or game	X	1	2	3	4	5	6
❏ Saw an upsetting TV show or movie, read an upsetting book, etc.	X	1	2	3	4	5	6

You will probably think of more sources of stress and things that upset you. Take your time. This could prove useful in helping you find a calmer outlook on life. This outlook will, in turn, help you change your behavior.

Causes of Stress	What I Can Do About Them

Worksheet 21B: What Can I Do Instead of Eating?

Put a check next to some of the things you could do instead of eating.

- ❏ Read a magazine or book that lets me escape into fantasy.
- ❏ Work on my favorite hobby. If I don't have one, begin to think of things that I like or would like to do.
- ❏ Call a friend or someone supportive.
- ❏ Take a soothing bath or a long, hot shower.
- ❏ Rent a movie, go to the movies or museum, see a play.
- ❏ Do some light cleaning. Organize drawers, do the dishes, or clean out a closet.
- ❏ Go for a walk outside, if it's nice. Change my scenery, and enjoy the fresh air.
- ❏ Exercise. Go to the gym, go for a walk, ride my bike, or go for a swim.
- ❏ Buy a small gift for myself or go window shopping.
- ❏ Put on my favorite song and dance around the room.
- ❏ Write a letter to someone I have not spoken to for a long time.
- ❏ Find a good low-calorie recipe that looks fun to prepare. Enjoy the creativity of preparing and cooking a healthy meal.
- ❏ (If you have a pet) Take my pet for a walk. Visit a pet store. (Pets are very comforting and give you a sense of calm and peacefulness.)
- ❏ Have a large glass of water. (If you are really hungry, the feeling won't go away. But remember, wait 20 minutes before you decide to eat. This will give you time to make a different decision if you are eating because of stress.)

If you checked fewer than 3 of these options, look at your lifestyle, and identify some other activities that you could do instead of eating.

Don't forget:

- Examine behavioral patterns
- Perspective, not panic
- Is it real hunger or just my appetite talking?
- Speak to a friend or spouse
- Exercise—it's good for you

CHAPTER TWENTY-TWO

In this chapter, you learn
- about binge eating and patterns
- how to establish regular eating patterns
- to cope with emotional upsets
- to deal with those who encourage you to eat
- about the assertive model
- how to manage your time

Worksheets to complete
- Am I Ready to Stop Bingeing?
- My Goals
- Problem Solving
- Dealing With Those Who Encourage Me to Eat
- How Assertive Am I?
- Managing My Time

Emotional Eating

People often eat large amounts of food in a relatively short time. While they are eating, they feel they cannot stop. This pattern of eating is called binge eating and is sometimes referred to as "stuffing your feelings."

Binge Eating and Patterns

Binge eating is more common than you might think. Sometimes your cravings or emotions get the best of you, and, in a flash, you are polishing off a huge helping of food. The problem develops when you put yourself down by saying, "I'm so awful, why did I do this?" Then a flood of negative feelings pushes you to consume more. The pattern looks like this.

Bingeing ➔ feeling guilty, fat, and out of control ➔
strict dieting ➔ feeling deprived ➔ bingeing

Binge eaters attempt to control their weight three ways:

1. Not eating for long periods
2. Avoiding certain foods
3. Not eating enough

Not Eating for Long Periods

Skipping meals can make you extremely hungry and may lead to overeating. Some people believe that if you skip a meal, you will lose weight. The opposite is true. A major way the body spends energy is by generating heat. This is called thermogenesis. To lose weight, you must expend energy. Your metabolism produces heat as it goes about its everyday cellular activities. When you eat, you boost your metabolism and burn more energy. You slow down your metabolism when you do not eat. So, by eating meals regularly, you keep your metabolism going and burn energy.

Avoiding Certain Foods

Do you have a list of "forbidden" foods? When most people try to lose weight, they decide they cannot have certain foods. Unfortunately, these are often their favorite foods, the ones they crave. There are no good or bad foods. There is room for every food in a well-balanced diet.

Not Eating Enough

After having snacked, grazed, or starved for many hours, a binge eater may sit down to a light meal of twigs and berries, a meal totally inadequate for the body's needs. Insatiable hunger is bound to hit soon, followed by overeating. This becomes a vicious cycle. Once you overeat, you punish yourself by restricting your eating. However, your body's natural need for nutrients will win out. You'll be really hungry, and that's when you'll probably overeat.

Binge eaters have a more difficult time with weight loss than regular overeaters. Binge eaters lose control and usually binge in reaction to emotional stress. Unrealistic, overly rigid eating standards set them up for failure. Skipping meals, avoiding favorite foods, and eating too little (so you are always hungry) may work when you are really motivated, but after a few days or an emotional upset, the deprivation is too much. Many people turn to food, especially forbidden food, when they are sad, angry, or frustrated. If you are hungry from too-strict eating habits, you may lose control and eat far more than you want or intend to.

Many times you crave a food you have tried to avoid. You decide to eat just a little. But then that little voice inside gets louder and says, "I don't care anymore. I've messed up now. I might as well eat it all."

If you think you might be a binge eater, fill out the brief questionnaire on the next page to see where you are in your attempt to change your eating patterns.

Worksheet 22A: Am I Ready to Stop Bingeing?

1. I don't want to change my style of eating. ❏ True ❏ False
2. I think about my bingeing but do not know what to do. ❏ True ❏ False
3. I think about my bingeing, but I have not made any plans to do anything about it. ❏ True ❏ False
4. I think about bingeing and plan to do something in the next month. ❏ True ❏ False
5. I have thought about bingeing and tried to do something within the past year but gave up. ❏ True ❏ False
6. I think about my bingeing and try to make some small changes. ❏ True ❏ False
7. I have already chosen an eating change. ❏ True ❏ False
8. I am able to avoid bingeing sometimes but not always. ❏ True ❏ False

Answers

If you answered true,

1. You are not ready to address the problem at this time. Read the emotional eating section of this workbook. Think about how you have tried to manage your weight. Then, retake the questionnaire to see if your views have changed.
2. You are eager to change your eating style but you do not know how. No need for alarm. You will find the tools in this workbook to help you begin changing your eating habits.
3. You are getting ready to change. Monitoring your eating behavior by keeping a journal will help you become motivated. It can help you see what to focus on. It can make you aware of your habits and show how your moods are related to eating.
4. You are beginning to change. Continue monitoring your eating habits and begin setting short-term minigoals. For example, you tell yourself, "Tomorrow there is an office party at a restaurant. I can eat in moderation, but I will be very careful with the bread basket." Then review your day and your actions.
5–8. Congratulations! You are on your way. You have already attempted to change or are changing your behavior. Reviewing your past attempts to lose weight and your triggers makes it easier for you to prevent a binge. Keep a journal and set a minigoal each week to increase control over your eating habits.

Establishing Regular Eating Patterns

You may have identified a pattern of chaotic eating. Everyone needs to establish realistic and regular eating patterns. In the past, your attempt to lose weight was probably focused on that dreaded four-letter word—diet.

As odd as it may seem, you will not be on a diet. Eating well does not have to mean depriving yourself. Instead, you are changing your mind-set. You are on your way to a healthier you. It's a lifetime process. You first must understand the way you think about things and how your self-talk gets you into trouble.

> To become aware, you need to examine
>
> - how much you eat
> - when you eat
> - what triggers your eating

Worksheet 22B: My Goals

In this section, you set some short-term goals for yourself. These are the kind of goals that lead to long-term success.

1. Weigh yourself only once a week. You punish yourself when you get on the scale every day because you can be upset by fluctuations. It is better to weigh yourself on the same day at the same time every week.

   I will weigh myself on _____ (day of the week)

2. Start eating three regular meals daily (breakfast, lunch, and dinner) and one or two planned snacks, either in late morning or late afternoon.

   This week for _____ days I will have three balanced meals and one or two snacks.

3. Stop counting calories or fat grams. Keep a daily food diary, but do not record calories. You are getting used to the idea that you are not dieting. Try to understand your feelings about eating and bingeing.

   This week I will keep a food diary without counting calories or fat grams. I'll record what I ate, when I ate it, and how I felt about it. I will do this for _____ days.

4. Moderation, not deprivation, is the goal. Choose one forbidden or problem food. Remember that trying to avoid your favorite foods can set you up for failure, because you will crave these foods. You can eat well without punishing yourself.

   This week I will add (how much) _____ of (forbidden food) _____ to my menu on (day of the week) _____.

Coping With Emotional Upsets

Stressful and upsetting feelings often may lead you to binge. You turn to food as a source of comfort, yet you realize this is a poor way to manage feelings. After you finish bingeing, you still have the feelings, but now they are accompanied by guilt and depression. While you were eating, you might have felt better, but it did not solve the original problem. What can you do to handle this?

Physical Activity

Activity is a truly effective way to reduce stress. You don't have to run every day or do step aerobics. Twenty minutes of walking a day can minimize stress and increase your stamina. Recruit a friend to go with you. Involve your family and become fit together.

Restructuring Your Thinking

When you restructure your thoughts, you change the way you view a situation. Often, your thoughts are distorted, pessimistic, and depressed. An inner voice can be either your enemy or your friend. Examine the ways you can begin to change your thinking.

1. Suppose you have had a lapse and binge. Where do you go from there? A lapse does not have to mean loss of control. You are not a failure. Think of the lapse as evidence of inadequate effort rather than inadequate ability. Remember, you can control what happens next.

2. View a lapse as part of the learning process, and use it. Slips are normal and to be expected.

3. A binge is a single event. Focus on it alone. What caused it? How can you prevent it? Do not say to yourself, "Uh oh, when this happened before, I really blew it." Avoid generalizing the situation.

4. Find an external (outside), specific, and controllable reason for the slip. Do not blame yourself for your inadequacies. Rather, look at it this way.
   - I was in a difficult, high-risk situation.
   - My coping skills were inadequate, but I am learning new ones.
   - For a moment, I lost my motivation. (I am tired, stressed…)
   - This is a situation I have not dealt with before.

Problem Solving

You need a general strategy for problem solving. This helps you break down overwhelming situations into manageable pieces.

To help you collect your energies, remember: S-O-D-A-S*

Stop
Options
Decide
Act
Self-praise

Stop and identify the problem.

Options—list all the possible solutions.

Decide which option is the best.

Act—Outline a step-by-step plan to put your decision into action.

Self-praise—Give yourself encouragement or pats on the back for solving your problem.

---

*The acronym SODAS was adapted by Maura Kirkham and colleagues [1986] as a strategy for problem solving. It originally appeared in Kirkham, MA, Schilling, RF, Norelius, K, Schinke, SP. Developing coping styles and social support networks: an intervention outcome study with mother of handicapped children. *Child: Care, Health and Development* 12: 313–323, 1986.

Worksheet 22C: Problem Solving

Use the following outline to practice this problem-solving technique. Although this exercise may seem corny, it will help you remember this coping mechanism.

1. **Stop!** What is the problem? _____

   _____

   _____

2. What are my **options** in solving this problem? _____

   _____

   _____

3. Which solution do I choose? _____

   _____

   _____

4. What **action** will I take to implement my **decision?** What are the steps? _____

   _____

   _____

5. What can I say to **pat** myself on the back? _____

   _____

   _____

6. I plan to use this problem-solving technique whenever...

   _____

   _____

Dealing With Those Who Encourage Me to Eat

Being assertive means standing up for yourself, but you don't have to be loud or mean to do it. Express your thoughts and feelings directly and appropriately. This increases your self-respect, as well as other people's respect for you. One of the major reasons for being assertive is to increase your control over yourself. There are times when you need to be assertive, especially when others are encouraging you to eat. Take a look at the following example.

You want to refuse an extra helping of food at a dinner party. What is the best thing for you to say?

a. You'd just love me to put on a few pounds of fat, wouldn't you?
b. Since you insist, I'll change my mind. I guess I'll have another piece.
c. It looks great, but I don't want any more, thank you.

C is correct. The answer may seem obvious on paper, but it is not always easy to assert yourself. The following worksheet helps you get better prepared to be assertive.

Worksheet 22D: Dealing With Those Who Encourage Me to Eat

What would you do in the following examples?

1. You buy some groceries at the supermarket, and after you leave, you discover that your change is a dollar short.

   I would _____

   _____

   _____

2. You order a rare steak at a restaurant, and it arrives well done.

   I would _____

   _____

   _____

3. You are waiting for a friend to get ready for work because you are driving. She is taking her time doing last-minute things. You are going to be late.

   I would _____

   _____

   _____

4. You are waiting in line at the deli, and someone pushes in front of you. The counter person does not notice and serves that person first.

   I would _____

   _____

   _____

5. A very close friend or family member asks you a difficult favor. You do not feel like doing it.

I would _____

_____

_____

6. You are at the movies, and the people behind you do not stop talking even after you've told them to be quiet.

I would _____

_____

_____

Answers

If you have a difficult time letting others know how you feel, you tend to be passive in your communication. You may be trying to avoid confrontation or conflict. However, in reality, you are giving a subtle message that you do not count. This is a pattern of nonassertiveness, and it makes it hard for you to get your needs met.

You may be passive-aggressive. Instead of openly dealing with an issue or person, you express angry feelings in a more hidden way. For example, instead of directly asking for what you want, you may continually complain about what is missing. In this type of communication, you often end up frustrating yourself and those around you.

When you absolutely feel you are right and others are wrong, you could be communicating aggressively. You may be able to express your feelings honestly, but you do it at the expense of others, hurting their feelings. Instead of asking directly for what you want, you demand it.

Another nonassertive style is being manipulative. You don't openly express your wants and desires. Instead, you create an atmosphere where you make others feel sorry for or guilty toward you. You send the message "poor me" or "I do everything." In this way, you get others to take care of you, but they may also resent you or get angry.

You may react to different situations with different styles of communication. The first step is to identify problem situations where you do not communicate effectively. Often in weight management, you are presented with difficult situations concerning food. They require you to be assertive and communicate directly to accomplish your goals and meet your needs. Doing this helps your self-esteem.

The Assertive Model

This model can help you express your feelings in a constructive way.

Being assertive is effectively stating your opinions and what you want without violating other people's rights. You believe that, "You and I may have our differences, but we are both entitled to express ourselves." Everyone is important. You are not demanding or commanding. Instead, you are direct and honest, which will gain you the respect you deserve.

Worksheet 22E: How Assertive Am I?

Answer the following questions by putting a check next to each statement that applies to you.

When do you experience problems in being assertive?
- ❏ Asking someone for help
- ❏ Expressing my opinion particularly when it is different from everyone else
- ❏ Responding to criticism that I feel is unfair or unjust
- ❏ Speaking up when everyone is looking at me, especially in a large group
- ❏ Receiving a compliment or giving one
- ❏ Having to take charge and assign tasks to others
- ❏ Saying no to someone offering food
- ❏ Handling someone who tries to make me feel guilty
- ❏ Being able to say something when a situation or person annoys me
- ❏ Negotiating for something I want or need
- ❏ Asking an authority figure for something that benefits me
- ❏ Protesting a rip-off

With whom do you have problems being assertive?
- ❏ People I work with or my boss
- ❏ My partner, spouse, or mate
- ❏ My parents
- ❏ Elderly people
- ❏ Children
- ❏ Salespeople, clerks, hired help
- ❏ Close or old friends
- ❏ Complete strangers
- ❏ A group of more than two

When you are not assertive, what have you been unable to accomplish?
- ❏ Getting approval for things I've done successfully
- ❏ Enlisting other's help for a particular job
- ❏ Receiving more attention or time with my partner
- ❏ Not having to be nice to everyone or in every situation
- ❏ Being able to speak up in an important situation or group
- ❏ Asking for things I deserve
- ❏ Having free time for myself
- ❏ Being comfortable with salespeople, clerks, or strangers
- ❏ Overcoming feelings of helplessness; the idea that nothing really changes
- ❏ Initiating new relationships of all kinds
- ❏ Not feeling resentful and angry toward others
- ❏ Being listened to, understood, and acknowledged

(This checklist was adapted from Bower, SA, Bower, GH. *Asserting Yourself.* Reading, MA: Addison-Wesley, 1976.)

Now look back at these checklists. Think about situations and people that create problems for you or make you uncomfortable. If you want to change your nonassertive behavior, try thinking about it in the following way.

Describe a problem situation. Be specific. Include

- the environment (setting)
- the person it involved (who)
- time of day (when)
- what bothered you about the situation
- how you would normally deal with it
- what fears you have about possible consequences if you are assertive
- your final goal

Here's an example of how to use this strategy with a problem situation.

My friend Sue **(who),** often speaks incessantly about her relationship problems **(what)** when we meet for lunch during a workday **(when and where).** I end up just sitting there pretending to be interested **(how I normally deal with it).** If I interrupt her monologue, I'm worried that she will think I don't care or that I'm selfish **(fear).** I would like to change the subject and talk about something that is going on in my life **(final goal).**

This is my situation. _____

_____

_____

_____

_____

_____

_____

The Assertive Model can help you express your feeling in a constructive way. You can say

When you (describe the other person's behavior),

I feel (describe how their behavior affects you and use feeling words such as sad, angry, frustrated, or confused).

I prefer / want / need (describe the desired change).

Here's an example of the Assertive Model.

When you push me to eat dessert, I feel uncomfortable. I feel like you are forcing me to eat. Right now, I need your support while I'm trying to lose weight.

Being assertive also establishes a pattern of respect for future meetings. When you express your needs, wants, and feelings, you show confidence, and others will respect that. Remember these tips.

- Define your goal in detail. Be direct in your request or refusal. Don't allow room for a possible misunderstanding. For example, instead of saying, "I'm cold," say, "Would you please turn up the heater."

- Use feeling words. Express your own likes and interests. Instead of using phrases such as *all people*, or *everyone*, say "I feel" and "I think."

- Be careful how you phrase your statement. Don't correct people's personality. Focus on their behavior and how it affects you. You should not criticize who they are, you should point out that what they do affects you. Instead of saying, "You are so selfish for not calling to tell me you'd be home late," you can say, "When you don't call to tell me you will be late, it bothers me. I start to worry about where you may be. Next time, please make sure you call."

- Let your body, face, and voice convey the same feeling as your words. Use eye contact, be open and relaxed. You are not attacking, you are expressing yourself.

- Speak up for yourself. Don't let others take advantage of you. You can say no without feeling guilty. Be persistent if you have to. If you are hesitant, you allow others to make decisions for you.

- Do not feel the need to defend yourself. It is not necessary to justify every opinion, thought, or feeling. Simply state, "That's how I feel." You are entitled to your feelings.

- Watch out for negative thinking. Do not decide that people do not like you or that they disapprove of you. Challenge the "shoulds" and "oughts" in your own head that prevent you from doing what you want to do. You are entitled to certain rights. The following is a list of your rights.

My Indisputable Rights

1. I have the right to put myself first sometimes.
2. I have the right to make mistakes and not always be perfect.
3. I have the right to my feelings, regardless of what they are.
4. I have the right to my opinions, convictions, values, and judgments.
5. I have the right to change my mind and choose a different path.
6. I have the right to ask for help.
7. I have the right not to take responsibility for someone else's actions.
8. I have the right to say no.
9. I have the right to spend time by myself. It does not mean I'm selfish.
10. I have the right to refuse a request or not do something.
11. I have the right to be acknowledged, respected, and receive recognition.
12. I have the right to be happy.
13. I have the right to negotiate for my needs and wants.

Time Management

We often feel there are not enough hours in a day or days in a week to do everything we have to do. Managing your time, then, becomes crucial to helping you manage your emotions. If you can handle your time, you make room for pleasure. Everyone perceives time differently. That's why it is possible to change our perceptions about how much time we really have. First, look at how we mismanage our precious time.

- **Confusion.** When you say you are wasting too much time, ask yourself on what? Think about where you want to go. What are you trying to accomplish? Only after you have defined a goal will you be able to manage your time and not be disorganized.

- **Indecision.** What should I do? People often get stuck when they take on too many tasks or when they do not enjoy any of them. Indecision may lead you to procrastinate and destroys your sense of free time. You feel you have something hanging over your head. You may not be able to decide because of stress, fear of failing or of making the wrong decision, or lack of interest and motivation.

- **Avoidance.** How many times do you get up from your desk to get another cup of coffee? Or pick up the phone? Avoiding work by doing irrelevant things or daydreaming is another way of wasting your time.

- **Perfectionism.** One of the most common reasons for not getting things done is perfectionism. You procrastinate because you think that if you cannot get it perfect, why start? You need to learn to stop this thinking and just begin!

Now that you have read about some common pitfalls in handling time, what do you do? It is important to become aware of your behavior so you can change it. It's time to take inventory.

We often feel stressed because many of the things we should do outweigh many of things we want to do. When you don't do things you should do, you may feel like a failure. Then you view challenging situations as stressful. You forget that life is meant to be enjoyed.

In the next exercise, think about all the things you do daily. Break down your day into small components, categorizing your activities as either shoulds or wants. By doing this, you will get a better understanding of how you use your time and where you can make changes.

Worksheet 22F: Managing My Time Example

Time To From	Activity	Want 1	2	3	Equal 4	5	6	Should 7
6:30–7:30am	Shower, dress, eat, get ready				X			
7:30–8:00am	Drive to work					X		
8:00–1:00pm	Do paperwork, conference			X				
1:00–2:00pm	Eat lunch alone and in peace	X						
2:00–5:30pm	Complete the day's work						X	
5:30–6:45pm	Drive home in traffic				X			
6:45–7:30pm	Watch the news and relax		X					
7:30–8:30pm	Eat dinner	X						
8:30–9:30pm	Take a walk with a friend	X						
9:00–10:00pm	Speak to relative on the phone						X	

On a scale from 1 to 10, today I felt _____

Instructions

People differ in how much time they spend doing wants and shoulds. Some of our activities are a mix of wants and shoulds, like going to a party we will enjoy but that is also a social obligation. Select a typical weekday and a typical weekend day. Use the form on the next page to fill in your activities.

Rate each activity when it occurs. Include the following:

1. When you begin and end each activity.
2. A brief description of each activity.
3. Want-should rating: 1 = total want, 7 = total should, 4 = equal mix of both. Remember this is a subjective rating. There is no right or wrong answer.
4. On a scale from 1 to 10 (10 being great), rate how you feel about the day.

Understanding how you balance wants and shoulds is important. When life becomes unbalanced and there are more shoulds than wants in your day, you may turn to food for comfort. If there is not enough pleasure in your life, then food may fill the empty place.

Managing My Time

Time To From	Activity	Rating Want 1	2	Equal 3	4	5	Should 6	7

On a scale from 1 (bad) to 10 (good), today I felt _____

You may photocopy this document for future use.

Now that you've analyzed your time, you can set some specific goals.

1. Set Your Priorities
- List tasks that need to be done in order of importance.
- Break these down into small manageable steps, and give yourself a realistic deadline.
- Reevaluate from time to time. Your goals may change.
- Keep a to-do list of short-term goals, ones that can be accomplished within that week.
- Keep a list of long-range goals.

2. Filter Out the Unimportant and Unrealistic Goals
- Choose who and what are important. Say no to the rest. You can't be everywhere and do everything at the same time.
- Examine why it may be difficult to turn down others' requests. Are you afraid you will not be liked? Do you have a need to be perfect?
- Play devil's advocate. Ask yourself, "What is the worst that could happen if I do not do it?"

3. Avoid Procrastination and Inefficiency
- Structure your time so that you reward every accomplishment. For example, "I will work 30 minutes straight, and then I will take a break."
- Alternate easy and fatiguing tasks to avoid burnout.
- Learn to delegate. Ask yourself why you cannot do it. Express your concerns to those you ask to help you.
- Learn your own rhythms. Each of us has a different work style. Learn to trust it. Some people work better under pressure, others don't. If it's effective, work with it, not against it.

Section Five

APPENDICES

Appendix A

Keeping a Food Diary

A food diary is a good tool to use when you are trying to lose weight. At first, you may feel that writing down everything you eat is too time consuming or too much of a bother. As you become more accustomed to using a food dairy, it will get easier and the information is really helpful.

This section contains food diary pages for counting calories or fat grams, following a meal plan, and controlling emotional eating. There is also a diary page for keeping track of your weekly totals. You may have chosen a monitoring method in chapter 6, but you can use any of the food diary pages. The examples provided here are just suggestions. Use the format that works best for you, and adapt the format to best suit your needs. You can photocopy these food diary pages or use your own paper. Note that the exercise you do is also recorded on the food diary.

Food Diary: Calorie/Fat Counting

The Calorie/Fat Counting Food Diary has three columns for you to complete.

- In the first column, record the foods and beverages you eat.
- In the center column, write the amount of the food and beverage.
- In the third column, write the number of calories or fat grams in that food and beverage. Add the total number of calories or fat grams and write the number at the bottom of the third column under Total.

Use as many pages as you need for each day, but start with a new page each day.

Food Diary: Calorie/Fat Gram Weekly Totals

Use your day-to-day totals of calories or fat grams to fill in the Weekly Totals Food Diary. For the day of the week, record your total calories or fat grams. You can see how close you come to your goals for each day that you keep a record.

Food Diary: Meal Plan

At the bottom of the Meal Plan Food Diary is a chart of suggested food exchanges for 1200-, 1500-, and 1800-calorie meal plans.

- For the plan you have chosen, write the number of exchanges for each food group in the Plan column.
- For each day, mark the number of servings that you ate in each food group.

You can compare the number of servings you ate to the number of servings your meal plan suggests.

Food Diary: Emotional Eating

The Emotional Eating Food Diary has five columns to complete. You might alternate the different Food Diary forms. Use calorie/fat counting one week and this one the next.

- In the first column, record what you have eaten.
- In the second column, write the time you consumed the food and beverage.
- In the third column, write about what was going on. For example, who you are with, where you are, what situation you are in.
- Record whether the food and beverage you have eaten is a Regular Meal (R), a Binge (B) or an Unplanned Meal (U) in the fourth column.
- In the final column, write how you felt before you ate each food/beverage or meal.

Food Diary: Calorie/Fat Counting

Name _____ Date _____

Meal/Snack	Amount	Calories/Fat Grams

Total _____

Food Diary: Calorie/Fat Counting Weekly Totals

	Total Calories	Total Fat Grams	Exercise Minutes	Exercise Type
Monday				
Tuesday				
Wednesday				
Thursday				
Friday				
Saturday				
Sunday				

Food Diary: Meal Plan

Name _____ Date _____

Food Groups	Plan	Mon	Tue	Wed	Thu	Fri	Sat	Sun
Starches								
Fruits								
Meat/meat substitutes								
Vegetables								
Fats								
Dairy								
Exercise Minutes								
Exercise Type								

1200 calorie	1500 calorie	1800 calorie
6 starches	7 starches	9 starches
2 fruits	3 fruits	3 fruits
4oz meat/meat substitutes	6 oz meat/meat substitutes	6 oz meat/meat substitutes
3 vegetables	3 vegetables	4 vegetables
less than 2 fats	less than 3 fats	less than 4 fats
2 dairy	2 dairy	2 dairy
+ free food	+ free food	+ free food

Food Dairy: Emotional Eating

Name _____ Date _____

Food and Beverage	Time	Context: Who, Where, Situation	R=Regular Meal B=Binge U=Unplanned Meal	Feelings Before Eating

Appendix B

Introduction to Meal Plans

The meal plans in this section are only samples. See a registered dietitian (RD) to design a meal plan that fits you—the foods you prefer and your lifestyle. Research shows that people who work through this workbook with the assistance of a health care professional, such as an RD or a nurse educator, are more successful at losing weight and keeping it off.

For menu items marked with a small number, we provide the recipe in Appendix C, pages 226–257. Each recipe has a corresponding number so you can find it easily.

The following are menu plans set at 1200, 1500, and 1800 calories. Calorie levels given here are approximate. Read labels and measure your serving sizes to help you stay on your target calorie level. Also, be sure to drink plenty of fluids (6–8 cups daily).

Here are some things to keep in mind.

1. Fruits and vegetables have no fat.
2. Your style of eating may not necessarily follow that of the meal plan. Eat according to your own eating style. Do try to eat at the same time every day. Try not to let more than 3 to 4 hours go by without eating. Otherwise you might feel so hungry that you eat more than you need.
3. Milk exchanges include skim, ½%, and 1% milk and milk products. Cheese is calculated as a meat exchange.
4. An average slice of bread usually has about 80 calories. You can have "light" breads with fewer calories (about 40 calories). If you prefer, you can have two slices of the "light" bread equaling 80 calories.

5. If you prefer vegetarian meals, substitute legumes (peas, lentils, and beans) for meats. Try peas, lentils, and beans in combination with corn or rice.
   - 1 cup cooked legume = 2 starch and 2 very lean meat
6. For meat substitutes you may use eggs, cottage cheese, skim milk cheeses, tofu, or soy beans. As dinner tends to be the meal where meat is most often used, try
   - pasta, beans, and cheese combination
   - rice and legumes
   - Mexican enchiladas and burritos with beans

1200-Calorie Sample Menu

Day One	Food Exchanges

Breakfast

½ cup shredded wheat cereal	1 starch
½ cup skim milk	½ milk
½ banana (9-inch)	1 fruit
coffee or tea with ½ cup skim milk	½ milk
and artificial sweetener	

Lunch

1 serving Chicken Rigatoni[1]	2 starch, 2 veg, 2 meat
1 slice whole wheat bread or	
7 melba toasts	1 starch
1 cup raw carrot sticks	1 veg

Dinner

½ serving Italian Grilled Tuna[2]	2 meat
1 serving Herb-Roasted Potatoes[28]	1 starch, 1 fat
1 dinner roll	1 starch
½ cup steamed broccoli	1 veg
1 cup green salad with balsamic vinegar	1 free food
1 serving Layered Vanilla Yogurt Parfaits[12]	1 fruit, ½ milk

Snack

1 Strawberry Milkshake[6]	1 fruit, 1 milk

Total: 6 starch, 3 fruit, 2½ milk, 4 veg, 4 meat, 1 fat, 1 free food
Total daily calories: 1250
Percent of total calories from fat: 18

1200-Calorie Sample Menu

Day Two	Food Exchanges

Breakfast

1 cup Country Cereal[7]	2 starch, 1 fruit
½ cup skim or 1% milk	½ milk
coffee or tea with ½ cup skim milk	
with artificial sweetener	½ milk

Lunch

1 sandwich (1 slice bread with 2 oz	1 starch
lean turkey or chicken or fish)	2 meat
1 Tbsp low-fat mayonnaise	1 fat
lettuce and tomato salad	1 veg
2 Tbsp nonfat dressing	1 free food
1 small tangerine	½ fruit

Dinner

1 serving Quick Chili[8]	2 meat, ½ starch
3 saltine-type crackers	½ starch
½ cup brown rice	1 starch
1 cup steamed carrots	2 veg
1 serving Sliced Mangoes and Papaya with Lime[26]	1½ fruit
6 almonds, chopped	1 fat

Snack

3 cups air-popped popcorn	1 starch
1 cup skim milk flavored with almond	
extract and noncaloric sweetener	1 milk

Total: 6 starch, 3 fruit, 2 milk, 3 veg, 4 meat, 2 fat, 1 free food
Total daily calories: 1225
Percent of total calories from fat: 22

Day Three	Food Exchanges

Breakfast

1 whole toasted English muffin	2 starch
2 tsp whipped butter	1 fat
1 cup cantaloupe sliced	1 fruit
Coffee or tea sweetened with artificial sweetener and ½ cup skim or 1% milk	½ milk

Lunch

1 serving Ensalada Catalana[9]	1 veg, ½ fat
2 oz low-fat mozzarella bread sticks	2 starch
15 fresh grapes	1 fruit
¼ cup low-fat cottage cheese	1 meat

Dinner

1 serving Chicken Dijon[10]	3 meat
½ cup noodles	1 starch
1 tsp whipped butter	½ fat
½ cup steamed broccoli and	
½ cup steamed carrots in	
1 tsp whipped butter	2 veg, ½ fat
1 cup romaine salad with balsamic vinegar	1 free food

Snack

1 cup skim milk	1 milk
4–6 crackers	1 starch
1 sliced apple	1 fruit

Total: 6 starch, 3 fruit, 1½ milk, 3 veg, 4 meat, 2½ fat, 1 free food
Total daily calories: 1205
Percent of total calories from fat: 16

1200-Calorie Sample Menu

Day Four	Food Exchanges
Breakfast	
1 slice toast with	1 starch
1 tsp butter or margarine	1 fat
8 oz fat-free, sugar-free yogurt	1 milk
coffee or tea with ½ cup skim milk	½ milk
and artificial sweetener	
½ cup orange juice	1 fruit
Lunch	
Salad bar:	
½ cup chickpeas	1 starch, 1 meat
1 cup lettuce	1 free food
1 cup raw carrots	1 veg
¼ cup mushrooms	1 free food
2 Tbsp balsamic vinegar	
1 slice bread or 5 melba toasts	1 starch
1 fresh apple	1 fruit
Dinner	
1 serving Mexican Beef Stir-Fry[16]	3 meat, 1 veg
½ cup Candied Yams[11]	1 starch
½ cup rice	1 starch
1 cup sliced tomatoes with balsamic vinegar	1 veg
1 tsp olive oil	1 fat
Snack	
1¼ cup strawberries topped with	1 fruit
½ cup nonfat plain yogurt	½ milk
3 (2½-inch square) graham crackers	1 starch

Total: 6 starch, 3 fruit, 2 milk, 3 veg, 4 meat, 2 fat, 2 free food
Total daily calories: 1225
Percent of total calories from fat: 22

1200-Calorie Sample Menu

Day Five	*Food Exchanges*

Breakfast

1 bagel	2 starch
2 tsp whipped butter or	
2 Tbsp reduced-fat cream cheese	1 fat
½ cup mango sliced or other fruit or	
½ cup fruit juice	1 fruit
coffee or tea with ½ cup skim milk	½ milk
with artificial sweetener	

Lunch

2 oz turkey with 1 tsp mayonnaise	2 meat, 1 fat
1 slice whole grain bread	1 starch
1 cup raw carrots	1 veg
1¼ cup watermelon or 5″ x 3½″ x 1″ wedge	1 fruit
1 cup green salad with balsamic vinegar	1 free food

Dinner

1 serving Cinnamon Chicken Salad[19]	3 meat, 1 veg
1 corn on the cob, boiled	1 starch
½ cup grilled zucchini (with nonstick spray)	1 veg
½ cup grilled eggplant (with nonstick spray)	1 veg
1 slice bread	1 starch
1 serving Layered Vanilla Yogurt Parfaits[12]	1 fruit, ½ milk

Snack

3 cups air-popped popcorn with chili powder	1 starch

Total: 6 starch, 3 fruit, 1 milk, 4 veg, 5 meat, 2 fat, 1 free food
Total daily calories: 1215
Percent of total calories from fat: 24

1200-Calorie Sample Menu

Day Six	*Food Exchanges*

Breakfast

1 bagel	2 starch
1 Tbsp fat-free cream cheese	1 free food
½ mango, sliced or ½ cup apple juice	1 fruit
coffee or tea with ½ cup skim milk with artificial sweetener	½ milk

Lunch

1 serving Orzo with Spinach and Feta Cheese[14]	2½ starch
1 cup Hellenic Village Salad[15]	1 veg, 1 fat
5 whole wheat fat-free crackers	1 starch
½ cup low-fat cottage cheese	2 meat

Dinner

½ serving Italian Grilled Tuna[2]	2 meat
2 servings Chinese Stir-Fried Vegetables[17]	2 veg, 1 fat
½ cup brown rice	1 starch
1 cup green salad with mustard and vinegar	1 free food
1 tsp olive oil	1 fat

Snack

8 oz nonfat plain yogurt with	1 milk
½ cup sliced fruit	1 fruit

Total: 6½ starch, 2 fruit, 1½ milk, 3 veg, 4 meat, 3 fat, 2 free food
Total daily calories: 1205
Percent of total calories from fat: 25

Day Seven	*Food Exchanges*

Breakfast

¾ cup cold cereal (unsweetened)	1 starch
½ cup skim or 1% milk	½ milk
1 cup coffee with ½ cup skim or 1% milk	½ milk
1 slice toast or ½ bagel	1 starch
1 Tbsp regular cream cheese	1 fat
½ banana (9-inch)	1 fruit

Lunch

1 serving Cinnamon Chicken Salad[19]	3 meat, 1 veg
1 serving Marinated Cucumbers[20]	1 veg
5 fat-free or whole grain crackers	1 starch
1 cup raw carrots	1 veg
1 medium peach	1 fruit

Dinner

1 serving Tortellini Salad[27]	1½ starch, 1 veg, ½ fat
2 Tbsp Parmesan cheese, grated	1 meat
1 cup red and green pepper salad with	1 veg
1 tsp olive oil	1 fat
1 serving Chocolate Angel Food Cake[21]	1 starch
2¼ Tbsp Berry Sauce[21]	1 free food

Snack

1 cup nonfat yogurt	1 milk

Total: 5½ starch, 2 fruit, 2 milk, 5 veg, 4 meat, 2½ fat, 1 free food
Total daily calories: 1198
Percent of total calories from fat: 25

1500-Calorie Sample Menu

Day One	**Food Exchanges**

Breakfast

1 cup shredded wheat cereal	2 starch
1 cup skim or 1% milk	1 milk
½ banana (9-inch)	1 fruit
Coffee or tea with ½ cup skim or 1% milk	½ milk

Lunch

1 serving Chicken Rigatoni[1]	2 starch, 2 veg, 2 meat
1 slice whole grain bread or roll	1 starch
with 1 tsp butter or margarine	1 fat
1 cup skim or 1% milk	1 milk

Dinner

1 serving Halibut in Foil[22]	4 meat
1 serving Herb-Roasted Potatoes[28]	1 starch, 1 fat
½ cup broccoli with lemon juice	1 veg
2 cups green salad with	
1 Tbsp nonfat salad dressing	3 free food
1 serving Fresh Apple Crisp[23]	2 fruit, 1 starch, 1 fat

Snack

¾ oz pretzels	1 starch

Total: 8 starch, 3 fruit, 2½ milk, 3 veg, 6 meat, 3 fat, 2 free food
Total daily calories: 1540
Percent of total calories from fat: 29

Day Two	*Food Exchanges*

Breakfast

1 cup Country Cereal[7]	2 starch, 1 fruit
½ cup skim or 1% milk	½ milk
1 cup coffee or tea with ½ cup skim milk	½ milk
½ cup orange juice	1 fruit

Lunch

1 sandwich (2 oz chicken)	2 meat
2 slices bread	2 starch
1 Tbsp reduced-fat mayonnaise	1 fat
1 cup raw carrots	1 veg
1 cup sliced tomatoes	1 veg

Dinner

2 cups Quick Chili[8]	4 meat, 1 starch
½ cup rice	1 starch
6 saltine-type crackers	1 starch
1 serving Sliced Mangoes and Papaya with Lime[26]	1½ fruit
2 servings Marinated Cucumbers[20]	2 veg
⅛ avocado, medium	1 fat

Snack

1 cup skim milk flavored with almond extract and noncaloric sweetener	1 milk
1 Tbsp nuts	1 fat

Total: 7 starch, 3½ fruit, 2 milk, 4 veg, 6 meat, 3 fat
Total daily calories: 1515
Percent of total calories from fat: 25

1500-Calorie Sample Menu

Day Three	*Food Exchanges*

Breakfast

2 slices toasted English muffin	2 starch
1 tsp butter	1 fat
1 cup cantaloupe	1 fruit
coffee or tea with ½ cup skim or 1% milk	½ milk

Lunch

Salad:

2 cups greens and fresh spinach	2 veg
1 oz sliced turkey	1 meat
1 oz low-fat Swiss cheese	1 meat
1 Tbsp regular salad dressing	1 fat
2 slices rye bread	2 starch
1 fresh pear	1 fruit
1 cup skim or 1% milk	1 milk

Dinner

1 serving Chicken Dijon[10]	3 meat
1 cup cooked noodles	2 starch
2 cups romaine salad with	
1 Tbsp nonfat salad dressing	2 free food
1 serving Ensalada Catalana[9]	1 veg, ½ fat
1 dinner roll	1 starch
1 tsp butter	1 fat

Snack

1 cup skim milk	1 milk
1 sliced apple	1 fruit

Total: 7 starch, 3 fruit, 2½ milk, 3 veg, 5 meat, 3½ fat, 2 free food
Total daily calories: 1473
Percent of total calories from fat: 26

Day Four	*Food Exchanges*

Breakfast

1 cup cooked oatmeal	2 starch
½ cup skim or 1% milk	½ milk
1 kiwi, peeled and sliced or ¼ cup raisins	1 fruit
coffee or tea with ½ cup skim or 1% milk	½ milk

Lunch

Salad bar:

1 oz lean ham	1 meat
1 cup chickpeas	2 starch, 2 meat
1 cup lettuce	1 free food
1 Tbsp sesame seeds	1 fat
1 cup raw carrots	1 veg
¼ cup mushrooms	1 free food
1 tsp balsamic vinegar and mustard	1 free food
1 tsp olive oil	1 fat
1 slice bread or 5 melba toasts	1 starch
1 fresh apple	1 fruit

Dinner

1 serving Mexican Beef Stir-Fry[16]	3 meat, 1 veg
1 slice bread or roll	1 starch
1 tsp butter or margarine	1 fat
½ cup rice with dill	1 starch
1 cup green salad with	
2 Tbsp reduced-fat salad dressing	1 free food, 1 fat
1 cup tomatoes with balsamic vinegar	1 veg, 1 free food

Snack

1¼ cup strawberries topped with	1 fruit
1 cup nonfat plain yogurt	1 milk

Total: 7 starch, 3 fruit, 2 milk, 3 veg, 6 meat, 4 fat, 5 free food
Total daily calories: 1505
Percent of total calories from fat: 27

1500-Calorie Sample Menu

Day Five	*Food Exchanges*

Breakfast

1 whole toasted English muffin	2 starch
1 tsp butter	1 fat
½ mango, sliced or ½ grapefruit	1 fruit
coffee or tea with ½ cup skim milk	½ milk

Lunch

3 oz turkey	3 meat
2 slices whole grain bread	2 starch
1 cup raw carrots	1 veg
1 pear	1 fruit
1 cup nonfat or 1% fat milk	1 milk

Dinner

½ cup vegetable juice	1 veg
1 serving Chicken Dijon[10]	3 meat
1 corn on the cob, boiled	1 starch
½ cup sliced grilled zucchini	1 veg
½ cup sliced grilled eggplant	1 veg
1 tomato, sliced	1 veg
1 serving Island Fruit Cup[24]	1 fruit
1 serving Brown Rice Pudding[13]	1½ starch

Snack

3 cups air-popped popcorn with chili powder or cinnamon	1 starch
1 tsp butter or margarine	1 fat

Total: 7½ starch, 3 fruit, 1½ milk, 5 veg, 6 meat, 2 fat
Total daily calories: 1460
Percent of total calories from fat: 23

1500-Calorie Sample Menu

Day Six	*Food Exchanges*

Breakfast

1 bagel	2 starch
2 Tbsp low-fat cream cheese	1 fat
½ cup pineapple or grapefruit segments	1 fruit
coffee or tea with ½ cup skim milk	½ milk

Lunch

1 serving Orzo with Spinach and Feta Cheese[14]	2½ starch
2 cups Hellenic Village Salad[15]	2 veg, 2 fat
5 whole-wheat fat-free crackers	1 starch
1 cup skim or 1% milk	1 milk

Dinner

1 serving Italian Grilled Tuna[2]	4 meat
2 servings Chinese Stir-Fried Vegetables[17]	2 veg, 1 fat
½ cup brown rice	1 starch
1 serving Roasted Potato and Carrot Salad[18]	1 starch, ½ fat
1 fresh nectarine	
or ½ cup canned fruit in juice	1 fruit

Snack

1 oz nonfat ricotta cheese	1 meat
15 grapes	1 fruit

Total: 7½ starch, 3 fruit, 1½ milk, 4 veg, 5 meat, 4½ fat
Total daily calories: 1495
Percent of total calories from fat: 28

1500-Calorie Sample Menu

Day Seven	*Food Exchanges*

Breakfast

1½ cups cold cereal (unsweetened)	2 starch
1 cup skim or 1% milk	1 milk
½ cup fruit salad	1 fruit
with 1 oz part-skim mozzarella cheese	1 meat

Lunch

2 servings Tropical Chicken Salad[29]	2 meat, 2 fruit, 1 fat
1 slice whole-grain bread or	
5 whole-grain fat-free crackers	1 starch
1 cup raw carrot and celery sticks	1 veg

Dinner

3 oz London Broil	3 meat
2 servings Tortellini Salad[27]	3 starch, 2 veg, 1 fat
1 cup green and red pepper salad	1 veg
1 serving Chocolate Angel Food Cake[21]	1 starch
2¼ Tbsp Berry Sauce[21]	1 free food

Snack

| 1 cup nonfat yogurt with mint | 1 milk |
| 4 walnut halves, crushed | 1 fat |

Total: 7 starch, 3 fruit, 2 milk, 4 veg, 6 meat, 3 fat, 2 free food
Total energy intake: 1485
Percent of total calories from fat: 25

1800-Calorie Sample Menu

Day One	*Food Exchanges*

Breakfast

2 shredded wheat biscuits	
or 1½ cups Cheerios	2 starch
1 cup skim or 1% milk	1 milk
1 cup coffee with artificial sweetener	1 free food

Lunch

1 serving Chicken Rigatoni[1]	2 starch, 2 veg, 2 meat
1 slice Italian bread	1 starch
1 tsp butter or margarine	1 fat
1 serving Fresh Apple Crisp[23]	2 fruit, 1 starch, 1 fat

Snack

| 1 Strawberry Milkshake[6] | 1 milk, 1 fruit |

Dinner

1 serving Halibut in Foil[22]	4 meat
1 cup rice	2 starch
1 cup cooked broccoli	2 veg
2 cups green salad	2 free food
1 Tbsp balsamic vinaigrette (1 tsp olive oil)	1 fat

Snack

1 cup skim milk with almond extract	
and artificial sweetener	1 milk
3 cups air-popped popcorn	1 starch
1 tsp butter or margarine	1 fat

Total: 9 starch, 3 fruit, 3 milk, 4 veg, 6 meat, 4 fat, 2 free food
Total daily calories: 1780
Percent of total calories from fat: 25

1800-Calorie Sample Menu

Day Two	*Food Exchange*

Breakfast

1 cup cooked cereal	2 starch
½ cup skim or 1% milk	½ milk
½ cup apple juice or ¼ cup raisins	1 fruit
½ cup skim or 1% milk with coffee	½ milk

Lunch

1 Sandwich:	
2 oz lean turkey or chicken	2 meat
2 slices bread	2 starch
1 tsp mayonnaise	1 fat
1 large sliced tomato and 1 cup raw carrots	2 veg
1 fresh orange, peach, or pear	1 fruit

Snack

1 cup plain nonfat yogurt with	1 milk
sliced cucumbers and dill	1 free food

Dinner

2 cups Quick Chili[8]	1 starch, 4 meat
6 saltine crackers	1 starch
1 cup white or brown rice	1 starch
1 cup broccoli cooked with	2 veg
1 tsp olive oil or margarine or butter	1 fat
½ banana (9-inch)	1 fruit
1 green salad with 1 tsp balsamic vinegar and	1 free food
1 tsp olive oil	1 fat

Snack

½ banana (9-inch)	1 fruit
1½ oz pretzels	2 starch

Total: 9 starch, 4 fruit, 2 milk, 4 veg, 6 meat, 3 fat, 2 free food
Total daily calories: 1785
Percent of total calories from fat: 23

1800-Calorie Sample Menu

Day Three	*Food Exchanges*

Breakfast
1 whole toasted English muffin	2 starch
with 2 tsp butter or margarine	2 fat
1 cup cantaloupe	1 fruit
coffee with ½ cup skim or 1% milk	½ milk

Lunch
Chef Salad:

2 oz ham or turkey	2 meat
1 hard-boiled egg, sliced	1 meat
1 oz low-fat cheese	1 meat
1 cup green and red peppers, sliced	1 veg
1 cup tomatoes, sliced	1 veg
2 cups lettuce	2 free food
2 Tbsp reduced-fat salad dressing	1 fat
2 slices rye bread	2 starch
2 tsp butter or margarine	2 fat
2 small plums	1 fruit

Dinner
1 serving Chicken Dijon[10]	3 meat
1 cup noodles	2 starch
1 cup green beans	2 veg
1 serving Chocolate Pudding[4]	1½ starch

Snack
1 cup skim milk	1 milk
4–6 crackers	1 starch
1 apple	1 fruit

Total: 9 starch, 3 fruit, 1½ milk, 4 veg, 7 meat, 5 fat, 2 free food
Total daily calories: 1785
Percent of total calories from fat: 29

1800-Calorie Sample Menu

Day Four	*Food Exchange*
Breakfast	
2 slices toast with	2 starch
2 Tbsp low-fat cream cheese	1 fat
1 cup fat-free, sugar-free yogurt	1 milk
1 cup melon	1 fruit
coffee or tea with ½ cup skim milk	½ milk
Lunch	
Salad bar:	
2 oz lean ham	2 meat
½ cup chickpeas	1 starch, 1 meat
1 cup lettuce	1 free food
½ cup cucumbers	1 free food
¼ cup low-fat cottage cheese	1 meat
2 cups carrots	2 veg
¼ cup mushrooms	1 free food
1 tsp balsamic vinegar and 1 tsp olive oil	1 fat
1 pear	1 fruit
1 slice whole-grain bread or roll	1 starch
Snack	
4 low-fat mini-muffins (1½-inch diameter)	2 starch
1 tsp butter	1 fat
½ cup skim or 1% low fat milk	½ milk
Dinner	
1 serving Mexican Beef Stir-Fry[16]	3 meat, 1 veg
2 slices bread or 2 rolls	2 starch
1 tsp butter	1 fat
½ cup grilled eggplant	1 veg
½ cup grilled zucchini	1 veg
1 cup green salad with	
2 Tbsp nonfat salad dressing	1 free food
1 apple or peach	1 fruit
Snack	
3 ginger snaps	1 starch

Total: 9 starch, 3 fruit, 2 milk, 5 veg, 7 meat, 4 fat, 4 free food
Total daily calories: 1770
Percent of total calories from fat: 26

1800-Calorie Sample Menu

Day Five	*Food Exchange*

Breakfast

1 whole toasted English muffin	2 starch
2 tsp butter or margarine	2 fat
1¼ cups strawberries	1 fruit
coffee or tea with ½ cup skim milk	½ milk

Snack

8 oz fat-free, sugar-free yogurt	1 milk
3 (2½-inch square) graham crackers	1 starch

Lunch

1 sandwich:	
3 oz turkey	3 meat
2 slices bread	2 starch
1 Tbsp low-fat mayonnaise	1 fat
½ cup cooked squash or 1 cup raw vegetables	1 veg
1¼ cups watermelon	1 fruit

Snack

3 cups air-popped popcorn with chili powder	1 starch
1 apple	1 fruit
1 cup skim or 1% milk	1 milk

Dinner

1 serving Cinnamon Chicken Salad[19]	3 meat, 1 veg
2 corn on the cob, boiled	2 starch
1 tsp butter or margarine	1 fat
1 cup grilled zucchini	2 veg
½ cup grilled eggplant	1 veg
2 cups green salad with	
1 Tbsp nonfat salad dressing	2 free food
½ cup Brown Rice Pudding[13]	1½ starch

Total: 9½ starch, 3 fruit, 2½ milk, 5 veg, 6 meat, 4 fat, 2 free food
Total daily calories: 1800
Percent of total calories from fat: 25

1800-Calorie Sample Menu

Day Six	*Food Exchanges*

Breakfast

1 bagel	2 starch
2 Tbsp low-fat cream cheese	l fat
1 cup nonfat or 1% fat milk	1 milk
½ cup pineapple or 1 cup melon in season	1 fruit
coffee or tea with ½ cup skim or 1% milk	½ milk

Lunch

1 cup pasta with ½ cup prepared, low-fat meat sauce	2 starch, 2 meat, 1 veg
2 Tbsp part-skim parmesan cheese	1 meat
1 orange	1 fruit
2 cups lettuce and 2 Tbsp fat-free Italian dressing	2 free food

Snack

10 fat-free whole-wheat crackers	2 starch
1 apple	1 fruit

Dinner

1 serving Italian Grilled Tuna[2]	4 meat
2 servings Herb-Roasted Potatoes[28]	2 starch, 2 fat
½ cup grilled eggplant	1 veg
1 cup grilled zucchini brushed with 1 tsp olive oil	2 veg 1 fat

Snack

5 Vanilla Wafers	1 starch
1 cup skim or 1% milk	1 milk

Total: 9 starch, 3 fruit, 2½ milk, 4 veg, 7 meat, 4 fat
Total daily calories: 1790
Percent of total calories from fat: 26

1800-Calorie Sample Menu

Day Seven	Food Exchange

Breakfast
1½ cups cold cereal	2 starch
1 cup skim or 1% milk	1 milk
1 apple	1 fruit

Lunch
1 sandwich:	
1 oz nonfat or low-fat cheese	1 meat
2 oz lean roast beef or turkey	2 meat
1 Tbsp low-fat mayonnaise and lettuce	1 fat, 1 free food
2 slices whole-grain bread	2 starch
1 cup nonfat or 1% yogurt	1 milk
1 serving Marinated Cucumbers[20]	1 veg

Snack
2 plums	1 fruit

Dinner
3 oz London Broil	3 meat
2 servings Tortellini Salad[27]	3 starch, 2 veg, 1 fat
2 cups green salad with	2 free food
balsamic vinegar or nonfat dressing, and	
1 tsp olive oil	1 fat
½ cup cooked broccoli	1 veg
½ cup cooked carrots	1 veg

Snack
Strawberry Milkshake[6]	1 fruit, 1 milk
4 Lorne Doone Cookies	1 starch

Total: 8 starch, 3 fruit, 3 milk, 5 veg, 6 meat, 3 fat, 3 free food
Total daily calories: 1815
Percent of total calories from fat: 22

Appendix C

Recipe Collection

1. Chicken Rigatoni • *Diabetic Meals In 30 Minutes—Or Less*, p. 159
2. Italian Grilled Tuna • *Flavorful Seasons Cookbook*, p. 248
3. Herbed Potatoes • *Diabetic Meals In 30 Minutes—Or Less*, p. 140
4. Chocolate Pudding • *How to Cook for People with Diabetes*, p. 181
5. Tropical Mango Mousse • *Flavorful Seasons Cookbook*, p. 101
6. Strawberry Milkshake • *Healthy HomeStyle Cookbook*, p. 169
7. Country Cereal • *Quick & Hearty Main Dishes*, p. 59
8. Quick Chili • *Diabetic Meals In 30 Minutes—Or Less*, p. 34
9. Ensalada Catalana • *How to Cook for People with Diabetes*, p. 99
10. Chicken Dijon • *Easy & Elegant Entrees*, p. 39
11. Candied Yams • *How to Cook for People with Diabetes*, p. 158
12. Layered Vanilla Yogurt Parfaits • *Diabetic Meals In 30 Minutes—Or Less*, p. 162
13. Brown Rice Pudding • *Great Starts & Fine Finishes*, p. 66
14. Orzo with Spinach and Feta Cheese • *Flavorful Seasons Cookbook*, p. 103
15. Hellenic Village Salad • *Healthy HomeStyle Cookbook*, p. 38
16. Mexican Beef Stir-Fry • *Diabetic Meals In 30 Minutes—Or Less*, p. 104
17. Chinese Stir-Fried Vegetables • *World-Class Diabetic Cooking*, p. 156
18. Roasted Potato and Carrot Salad • *Flavorful Seasons Cookbook*, p. 195
19. Cinnamon Chicken Salad • *How to Cook for People with Diabetes*, p. 141
20. Marinated Cucumbers • *Southern-Style Diabetic Cooking*, p. 53
21. Chocolate Angel Food Cake with Berry Sauce • *World-Class Diabetic Cooking*, p. 178, p. 197
22. Halibut in Foil • *Diabetic Meals In 30 Minutes—Or Less*, p. 77
23. Fresh Apple Crisp • *Flavorful Seasons Cookbook*, p. 393
24. Island Fruit Cup • *How to Cook for People with Diabetes*, p. 96
25. Orange Mint Slaw • *How to Cook for People with Diabetes*, p. 37
26. Sliced Mangoes and Papaya with Lime • *Flavorful Seasons Cookbook*, p. 205
27. Tortellini Salad • *Brand-Name Diabetic Meals in Minutes*, p. 35
28. Herb-Roasted Potatoes • *Flavorful Seasons Cookbook*, p. 63
29. Tropical Chicken Salad • *Flavorful Seasons Cookbook*, p. 198

Chicken Rigatoni

Diabetic Meals In 30 Minutes—Or Less, p. 159

6 servings/serving size: 2 oz chicken with 1 cup pasta

1 Tbsp olive oil
12 oz boneless, skinless chicken breasts, cubed
1 medium onion, chopped
1 green pepper, seeded, cored, and cut into match stick strips
1 15-oz jar marinara sauce
Fresh ground pepper to taste
6 cups cooked rigatoni pasta

1. To prepare the sauce, heat the oil in a large skillet over medium heat. Add the chicken and sauté until chicken is no longer pink. Remove from the skillet.
2. In the remaining pan juices, sauté the onion and pepper. Add the cooked chicken to the skillet and add the marinara sauce. Grind in pepper.
3. Let the sauce simmer for about 5 minutes. Pour over the rigatoni and serve.

Starch Exchange	2
Lean Meat Exchange	2
Vegetable Exchange	2
Calories	312
Calories from Fat	62
Total Fat	7 g
Saturated Fat	2 g
Cholesterol	35 mg
Sodium	284 mg
Total Carbohydrate	41 g
Dietary Fiber	4 g
Sugars	6 g
Protein	19 g

Italian Grilled Tuna

Flavorful Seasons Cookbook, p. 248

6 servings/serving size: 3–4 oz

1½ lb tuna steaks
2 Tbsp fresh lemon juice
½ cup diced roasted red peppers
½ cup sliced scallions
2 Tbsp minced fresh oregano
2 Tbsp minced fresh Italian parsley
⅓ cup balsamic vinegar
1 Tbsp olive oil
Fresh ground pepper and salt to taste

1. Combine the tuna steaks and lemon juice and marinate for 15 minutes. Prepare an outside grill with an oiled rack set 6 inches above the heat source. On a gas grill, set the heat to medium.
2. Grill or broil the tuna 6 inches from the heat source for 4–5 minutes on each side. Combine all remaining ingredients in a saucepan and bring to a boil. Pour the sauce over the tuna steaks to serve.

Lean Meat Exchange	4
Calories	237
Calories from Fat	94
Total Fat	10 g
Saturated Fat	3 g
Cholesterol	69 mg
Sodium	52 mg
Total Carbohydrate	3 g
Dietary Fiber	0 g
Sugars	2 g
Protein	25 g

Diabetic Meals In 30 Minutes—Or Less, p. 140

6 servings/serving size: ½ cup

1½ lb small red potatoes
1½ tsp olive oil
6 sprigs rosemary
6 sprigs thyme
2 Tbsp white wine
2½ tsp paprika

1. Preheat the oven to 400° F. Wash and scrub the potatoes. Cut each potato in half.
2. Place about ½ cup of potatoes on 6 squares of foil large enough to fold over. Divide the olive oil, herbs, wine, and paprika evenly over each packet. Seal the packets and place in the oven.
3. Bake for 30 minutes. Let cool for 5 minutes. Place a packet on each plate and let each person carefully open the packet.

Starch Exchange	1½
Calories	110
Calories from Fat	11
Total Fat	1 g
Saturated Fat	0 g
Cholesterol	0 mg
Sodium	6 mg
Total Carbohydrate	23 g
Dietary Fiber	2 g
Sugars	2 g
Protein	2 g

Chocolate Pudding

4

How to Cook for People with Diabetes, p. 181

4 servings/serving size: ¼ recipe

2 Tbsp cornstarch
2 Tbsp unsweetened cocoa powder
¼ cup sugar
2 cups skim milk
1 tsp vanilla
¼ tsp other extract, such as rum, almond, or orange, if desired

1. In a medium saucepan, combine the cornstarch, cocoa powder, and sugar. Mix well. Gradually add the milk, stirring to dissolve the cornstarch and cocoa into the milk. Place over medium heat.
2. Continue cooking over medium heat, stirring until the mixture comes to a boil. Continue boiling the mixture for 2–3 minutes, stirring constantly.
3. Remove from the heat and stir in the vanilla and other extract, if desired. Spoon the pudding into 4 custard cups.

Starch Exchange	1½
Calories	109
Calories from Fat	5
Total Fat	1 g
Saturated Fat	0 g
Cholesterol	2 mg
Sodium	64 mg
Total Carbohydrate	23 g
Dietary Fiber	1 g
Sugars	17 g
Protein	5 g

Tropical Mango Mousse

Flavorful Seasons Cookbook, p. 101

6 servings/serving size: ½ cup

This light dessert can also be made with berries.

2 small mangoes, peeled and cubed
1 medium banana, peeled
⅔ cup plain nonfat yogurt
2 tsp honey
6 large ice cubes
1 tsp vanilla

In a blender, combine all ingredients until smooth. Refrigerate for 3 hours. Pour into individual dishes and serve.

Fruit Exchange	1½
Calories	87
Calories from Fat	3
Total Fat	0 g
Saturated Fat	0 g
Cholesterol	1 mg
Sodium	23 mg
Total Carbohydrate	21 g
Dietary Fiber	2 g
Sugars	18 g
Protein	2 g

Strawberry Milkshake

Healthy HomeStyle Cookbook, p. 169

1 12-oz serving

1 cup skim milk
½ ripe banana, peeled and sliced
3–5 ripe strawberries, hulls removed

1. Blend all ingredients in blender or food processor.
2. Double the recipe for 2 big shakes.

Skim Milk Exchange	1
Fruit Exchange	1
Calories	156
Calories from Fat	0
Total Fat	0 g
Saturated Fat	0 g
Cholesterol	0 mg
Sodium	125 mg
Total Carbohydrate	30 g
Dietary Fiber	3 g
Sugars	2 g
Protein	9 g

Quick & Hearty Main Dishes, p. 59

6 servings/serving size: ½ cup

2 cups skim milk
½ cup raisins
1 tsp cinnamon
3 cups precooked brown rice
2 strawberry halves per serving
1–1½ tsp pure maple syrup per serving

1. In a medium saucepan over medium heat, combine milk, rice, raisins, and cinnamon. Bring mixture to a boil, stirring occasionally. Reduce heat; cover and simmer for 8 to 10 minutes or until mixture thickens.
2. Spoon cereal into bowls, top with strawberries and syrup, and serve.

Starch Exchange	2
Fruit Exchange	1
Calories	206
Calories from Fat	11
Total Fat	1 g
Saturated Fat	0 g
Cholesterol	1 mg
Sodium	50 mg
Total Carbohydrate	44 g
Dietary Fiber	3 g
Sugars	20 g
Protein	6 g

Quick Chili

Diabetic Meals In 30 Minutes—Or Less, p. 34

6 servings/serving size: 1 cup

2 tsp olive oil
1 medium onion, chopped
1 small red pepper, chopped
4 cloves garlic, minced
1 lb lean pork tenderloin, trimmed and ground (your butcher will do this for you)
3 Tbsp ground chili powder
1 tsp cinnamon
½ tsp allspice
2 cups canned tomatoes, coarsely chopped, undrained
2 cups low-sodium beef broth
1 Tbsp red wine
1 Tbsp Worcestershire sauce
Fresh ground pepper to taste

1. In a stock pot over medium-high heat, heat the oil. Add the onion and pepper and sauté for 5 minutes. Add the garlic and sauté for 2 minutes. Add the pork and sauté for 5 minutes.
2. Add the remaining ingredients and simmer over medium-low heat for 20 minutes.

Lean Meat Exchange	2
Starch Exchange	½
Calories	160
Calories from Fat	53
Total Fat	6 g
Saturated Fat	1 g
Cholesterol	44 mg
Sodium	262 mg
Total Carbohydrate	11 g
Dietary Fiber	3 g
Sugars	5 g
Protein	18 g

How to Cook for People with Diabetes, p. 99

18 servings/serving size: ½ cup

1 medium eggplant
3 medium green peppers
3 medium onions
3 medium tomatoes
2 7-oz cans artichoke hearts
6 tsp olive oil
2 cloves garlic, minced
¼ cup chopped parsley
2 Tbsp capers in vinegar
⅛ tsp white pepper
¼ tsp salt
2 lemons
1 hard-boiled egg

1. Preheat the oven to 300° F. Place the eggplant, green pepper, onion, and tomatoes in a covered dish and roast for 60 minutes. Allow the vegetables to cool to room temperature, then peel and remove all seeds. Slice the vegetables into strips and add the artichoke hearts. Set aside.

2. Heat 1 tsp of the olive oil in a small skillet and sauté the garlic for 3–4 minutes. Add the parsley, capers, pepper, and salt. Squeeze the lemons and add the juice to the remaining oil. Mix this well with the garlic; then pour over the vegetables. Toss gently to coat and refrigerate before serving. Garnish with sliced egg.

Vegetable Exchange	1
Fat Exchange	½
Calories	51
Calories from Fat	18
Total Fat	2 g
Saturated Fat	0 g
Cholesterol	15 mg
Sodium	58 mg
Total Carbohydrate	8 g
Dietary Fiber	1 g
Protein	2 g

Chicken Dijon

Easy & Elegant Entrees, p. 39

8 servings/serving size: 3–4 oz

4 whole boneless, skinless chicken breasts, halved
1 Tbsp olive oil
¼ cup onion, minced
2 cups fresh mushrooms, sliced
2 cloves garlic, minced
½ cup low-sodium chicken broth
¼ cup dry white wine
Fresh ground pepper
4 Tbsp fresh parsley, minced
1 Tbsp Dijon mustard

1. Place chicken breasts between 2 sheets of waxed paper; flatten to ¼ inch using a meat mallet. Coat a large skillet with nonstick cooking spray and place over medium-high heat; heat until hot.
2. Add chicken to the skillet and cook for 2–3 minutes until chicken is browned on each side. Remove chicken from skillet; set aside and keep warm.
3. In the same pan, add the olive oil. sauté the onion, mushrooms, and garlic for 2–3 minutes. Add the wine, chicken broth, and 2 Tbsp of the parsley and cook for 3–4 minutes.
4. Add the chicken to the pan again and cook over medium heat for 10–12 minutes. Remove the chicken and vegetables using a slotted spoon. Arrange the chicken on a serving platter and keep warm.
5. Continue cooking broth mixture until it is reduced to ⅓ cup. Remove from heat; whisk in the remaining parsley and mustard. Spoon sauce over the chicken and serve.

Lean Meat Exchange	3
Calories	173
Calories from Fat	45
Total Fat	5 g
Saturated Fat	1 g
Cholesterol	72 mg
Sodium	93 mg
Total Carbohydrate	2 g
Dietary Fiber	1 g
Sugars	1 g
Protein	27 g

Candied Yams

How to Cook for People with Diabetes, p. 158

12 servings/serving size: ¼ cup

6 medium yams, boiled in skin until tender (about 20–30 minutes)
⅓ cup raisins
1 Tbsp brown sugar
3 Tbsp sugar substitute
2 tsp cinnamon
½ tsp nutmeg
Ground cloves to taste
⅓ cup low-calorie margarine
1 cup cold water

1. Preheat the oven to 350° F. Cool yams, peel, and slice lengthwise. Place the yam slices in a covered baking dish. Sprinkle the raisins over the yams.
2. In a separate bowl, mix the brown sugar, sugar substitute, and spices; sprinkle over the yams. Dot with margarine and add water.
3. Cover the baking dish and bake for 30 minutes. Remove the cover, then bake another 15–20 minutes.

Starch Exchange 1
Calories 81
    Calories from Fat.................22
Total Fat................................2½ g
Cholesterol ....0 mg
Sodium...............................63 mg
Total Carbohydrate ....14 g
    Dietary Fiber ....0 g
Protein ....1 g

Layered Vanilla Yogurt Parfaits

12

Diabetic Meals In 30 Minutes—Or Less, p. 162

6 servings/serving size: ½ cup yogurt with ½ cup fruit

3 cups plain nonfat yogurt
2 tsp vanilla extract
3 tsp fructose
1 banana, sliced
1 cup green grapes, halved
1 cup strawberries, sliced
¼ cup Grapenuts cereal

1. In a small bowl, combine the yogurt, vanilla, and fructose. Place a layer of the yogurt mixture in parfait, wine, or champagne glasses.
2. In another bowl, combine the fruits. Add a layer of fruit on top of the yogurt. Continue layering the yogurt and fruit until each glass has three layers, ending with yogurt.
3. Top each parfait with a sprinkle of Grapenuts cereal. Chill until ready to serve.

Fruit Exchange	1
Skim Milk Exchange	½
Calories	126
Calories from Fat	3
Total Fat	0 g
Saturated Fat	0 g
Cholesterol	3 mg
Sodium	129 mg
Total Carbohydrate	25 g
Dietary Fiber	2 g
Sugars	19 g
Protein	8 g

238 APPENDICES

Brown Rice Pudding

Great Starts & Fine Finishes, p. 66

10 servings/serving size: ½ cup

3 egg whites
1½ cups skim milk
2 tsp fructose
1 tsp vanilla
1 tsp lemon peel
2 tsp lemon juice
1 tsp cinnamon
½ tsp nutmeg
2 medium apples or pears, chopped
½ cup raisins
2 cups cooked brown rice

1. Preheat oven to 325° F. Beat together the egg whites, skim milk, and fructose.
2. Stir in the remaining ingredients. Pour the rice mixture into a baking dish and bake for 50 minutes or until set. Serve warm or cold.

Starch Exchange	1½
Calories	105
Calories from Fat	5
Total Fat	1 g
Saturated Fat	0 g
Cholesterol	1 mg
Sodium	38 mg
Total Carbohydrate	22 g
Dietary Fiber	2 g
Sugars	11 g
Protein	4 g

Flavorful Seasons Cookbook, p. 103

6 servings/serving size: ½ cup

1½ cups dry orzo
2 tsp olive oil
1 medium onion, minced
1 10-oz package frozen chopped spinach, thawed and well drained
¼ cup crumbled feta cheese
Fresh ground pepper to taste

1. Cook the orzo according to package directions. Drain.
2. Heat the oil in a skillet over medium-high heat. Add the onion and sauté for 5 minutes. Add the spinach and sauté for 4 more minutes.
3. Toss the onion-spinach mixture with the hot orzo. Add the feta cheese and ground pepper, and toss well. Serve immediately.

Starch Exchange	2½
Calories	204
Calories from Fat	30
Total Fat	3 g
Saturated Fat	1 g
Cholesterol	4 mg
Sodium	82 mg
Total Carbohydrate	37 g
Dietary Fiber	2 g
Sugars	4 g
Protein	8 g

Hellenic Village Salad

Healthy HomeStyle Cookbook, p. 38

8 servings/serving size: 1 cup

4–5 firm ripe tomatoes, sliced
1 clove garlic, cut
1 large cucumber, diced
2 medium green bell peppers, seeded and sliced
3 scallions or 1 round onion, sliced
16 Greek olives, rinsed
2 oz feta cheese, broken into small chunks
1 Tbsp olive oil
2 Tbsp vinegar
Fresh ground pepper
Dried oregano for garnish

1. Place the tomatoes in a salad bowl that has been rubbed with the cut garlic.
2. Add the cucumber, peppers, onions, olives, and feta.
3. Sprinkle the olive oil, vinegar, and pepper over the salad. Stir thoroughly. Top with oregano. Serve cold.

Vegetable Exchange	1
Fat Exchange	1
Calories	103
Calories from Fat	63
Total Fat	7 g
Saturated Fat	2 g
Cholesterol	6 mg
Sodium	414 mg
Total Carbohydrate	7 g
Dietary Fiber	2 g
Protein	3 g

Mexican Beef Stir-Fry 16

Diabetic Meals In 30 Minutes—Or Less, p. 104

6 servings/serving size: 3–4 oz

1 Tbsp canola oil
1½ lb lean sirloin steak, cut into 3-inch strips, trimmed of all fat
3 cloves garlic, minced
1 medium onion, minced
1 small red pepper, cut into thin strips
2 tsp chili powder
2 Tbsp lime juice
1 tsp cumin

1. In a wok over medium-high heat, heat the oil. Add the beef and sauté until the beef loses its pinkness. Drain any accumulated fat. Remove the beef from the wok.
2. Add the garlic and onions and sauté for 5 minutes. Add the red pepper and sauté for 5 more minutes.
3. Add the chili powder and lime juice to coat the vegetables. Add the beef back to the skillet and add the cumin. Heat 1 minute more.

Lean Meat Exchange	3
Vegetable Exchange	1
Calories	180
Calories from Fat	67
Total Fat	7 g
Saturated Fat	2 g
Cholesterol	65 mg
Sodium	58 mg
Total Carbohydrate	4 g
Dietary Fiber	1 g
Sugars	3 g
Protein	23 g

World-Class Diabetic Cooking, p. 156

6 servings/serving size: ¼ of recipe

Sauce
2 Tbsp cold water
1 Tbsp cooking sherry
2 tsp lite soy sauce
1 tsp cornstarch

Vegetables
1 tsp butter
1 tsp olive oil
1 onion, coarsely chopped
2 stalks celery, diagonally sliced
1 cup fresh cauliflower florets
1 cup fresh broccoli florets
½ cup chicken broth or water
2 Tbsp red sweet pepper or fresh parsley, finely chopped
Salt and fresh ground pepper

1. Sauce: In small dish or cup, combine water, sherry, soy sauce, and cornstarch. Mix well.
2. In large nonstick skillet or wok, heat butter and olive oil over medium-high heat. Stir-fry onion and celery for 4 minutes. Add cauliflower and broccoli; stir-fry for 4 minutes longer. Stir in broth, cover, and steam for 1 minute.
3. Push vegetables to one side. Stir sauce mixture into pan juices. Cook, stirring for 1 minute or until thickened. Fold into vegetables to lightly coat them. Stir in red pepper. Season to taste with salt and pepper. Serve immediately.

More Stir-Fry combinations:
Celery, onion, Bok choy or cabbage, red sweet pepper
Celery, onion, zucchini, mushrooms, red sweet pepper

You may add one or more of the following:
1 clove garlic, minced
1 Tbsp fresh ginger root, grated
1 Tbsp lemon or orange rind, shredded
a few grains of cayenne or crushed red chili peppers

Vegetable Exchange	1
Fat Exchange	½
Calories	42
Calories from Fat	18
Total Fat	2 g
Saturated Fat	0 g
Cholesterol	1 mg
Sodium	146 mg
Total Carbohydrate	5 g
Protein	2 g

Roasted Potato and Carrot Salad

Flavorful Seasons Cookbook, p. 195

6 servings/serving size: ½ cup

1½ cups red potatoes, unpeeled, diced
1½ cups carrots, thickly sliced
4 shallots, minced
3 cloves garlic, minced
1 Tbsp lemon juice
2 Tbsp olive oil
1 cup dry white wine
1 tsp cumin
Romaine lettuce leaves

1. Place all ingredients except the lettuce in a large roasting pan. Toss lightly to coat the vegetables well and roast, covered, for 45–60 minutes until the potatoes and carrots are very tender.
2. Remove the vegetables from the oven and chill. To serve, place the lettuce in a large salad bowl or platter and top with the roasted vegetables.

Starch Exchange	1
Monounsat Fat Exchange	½
Calories	107
Calories from Fat	41
Total Fat	5 g
Saturated Fat	1 g
Cholesterol	0 mg
Sodium	31 mg
Total Carbohydrate	14 g
Dietary Fiber	3 g
Sugars	3 g
Protein	2 g

Cinnamon Chicken Salad

19

How to Cook for People with Diabetes, p. 141

6 servings/serving size: 1 cup

¼ cup low-calorie mayonnaise
¼ cup nonfat plain yogurt
¾ tsp cinnamon
⅛ tsp cloves
⅛ tsp pepper
¼ tsp salt
1½ lb boneless, skinless, cooked chicken breast, diced
½ cup celery, diced
2 Tbsp toasted slivered almonds
1 cup seedless grapes, halved

1. In a small bowl, whisk the mayonnaise, yogurt, cinnamon, cloves, pepper, and salt together.
2. Put the remaining ingredients in a large bowl and add the mayonnaise dressing. Toss well and refrigerate before serving.

Vegetable Exchange	1
Lean Meat Exchange	3
Calories	202
Calories from Fat	72
Total Fat	8 g
Saturated Fat	1 g
Cholesterol	64 mg
Sodium	247 mg
Total Carbohydrate	5 g
Dietary Fiber	2 g
Sugars	14 g
Protein	26 g

246 APPENDICES

Southern-Style Diabetic Cooking, p. 53

6 servings/serving size: ²⁄₃ cup

4 cups cucumbers, thinly sliced
1 large onion, thinly sliced and separated into rings
1 cup water
1 cup vinegar, plain or flavored
1 tsp celery seed
½ tsp garlic powder (or 1 Tbsp fresh garlic, chopped)
½ tsp salt

1. If the cucumbers are waxed, peel them before slicing. If they are not waxed and are chemical-free, leave the skin on. With a fork, score the sides of each cucumber, creating a ruffled edge. Slice thinly.
2. Layer the sliced cucumbers and onion in a large bowl. Combine the remaining ingredients and blend thoroughly. Pour the dressing over the cucumbers. Cover and chill at least 2 hours. Use a slotted spoon to serve.

Vegetable Exchange	1
Calories	28
Calories from Fat	1
Total Fat	0 g
Saturated Fat	0 g
Cholesterol	0 mg
Sodium	100 mg
Total Carbohydrate	7 g
Dietary Fiber	1 g
Sugars	5 g
Protein	1 g

World-Class Diabetic Cooking, p. 178

1 angel food cake, 16 servings/serving size: $^1/_{16}$ of recipe

1½ cups egg whites (approximately 12), at room temperature
¼ cup water
1 tsp cream of tartar
½ tsp salt
1 cup granulated sugar
¾ cup cake and pastry flour, sifted
¼ cup unsweetened cocoa powder
1 tsp vanilla

1. In mixer bowl, beat egg whites, water, cream of tartar, and salt until frothy. Gradually add ¾ cup sugar and continue beating just until stiff, shiny peaks form and sugar is dissolved. (A bit of the mixture feels smooth when squashed between finger and thumb.)
2. In another bowl, lightly combine flour, cocoa, and remaining sugar. Sift over egg white mixture in 3 batches, and after each addition, with wire whisk, fold in until there are no little lumps of flour.
3. Spoon into ungreased 10-inch tube pan. With knife, cut through batter to remove bubbles. Smooth top.
4. Bake in 350° F oven for 50 minutes or until a cake tester comes out clean and the top springs back when lightly touched.
5. Invert pan, allowing cake to hang upside down on its own stand or funnel for at least 1 hour to cool. With sharp knife, loosen around edge; transfer to cake plate.

Carbohydrate Exchange	1
Calories	83
Calories from Fat	0
Total Fat	0 g
Saturated Fat	0 g
Cholesterol	0 mg
Sodium	111 mg
Total Carbohydrate	17 g
Dietary Fiber	0 g
Protein	3 g

Berry Sauce

World-Class Diabetic Cooking, p. 197

1¾ cups, 12 servings/serving size: 2¼ Tbsp

2 cups raspberries, blueberries, saskatoons, or blackberries
1 tsp lemon juice
Sugar substitute equivalent to ⅓ cup sugar

1. In food processor or blender, combine strawberries, lemon juice, and sugar substitute. Process until sauce-like. Drain liquid off of frozen berries before puréeing them to prevent the sauce from being too watery.

Free Food	1
Calories	12
Calories from Fat	0
Total Fat	0 g
Saturated Fat	0 g
Cholesterol	0 mg
Sodium	0 mg
Total Carbohydrate	3 g
Dietary Fiber	0 g
Protein	0 g

Diabetic Meals In 30 Minutes—Or Less, p. 77

6 servings/serving size: 3–4 oz

2 tsp olive oil
6 4-oz halibut steaks
½ cup dry white wine
6 thyme sprigs
6 thin lemon slices
1½ tsp fennel seeds
6 parsley sprigs
Fresh ground pepper to taste

1. Preheat the oven to 350° F. Tear aluminum foil into 6 large squares. Brush each square with some olive oil.
2. Place the halibut in the center of the square. Drizzle each steak with some of the wine. Put a thyme sprig, lemon slice, a few fennel seeds, and a parsley sprig on each piece of fish.
3. Grind pepper over each piece of fish. Seal the foil into a packet. Place all packets on a baking sheet and bake for 10–15 minutes. Place a packet on each plate and let each person carefully open the packet. Pour all juices on top of the fish.

Very Lean Meat Exchange	4
Calories	144
Calories from Fat	37
Total Fat	4 g
Saturated Fat	1 g
Cholesterol	36 mg
Sodium	62 mg
Total Carbohydrate	0 g
Dietary Fiber	0 g
Protein	24 g

Fresh Apple Crisp

Flavorful Seasons Cookbook, p. 393

6 servings/serving size: 1 medium apple with ¼ cup topping

6 medium Granny Smith apples, unpeeled and sliced
2 Tbsp fresh lemon juice
2 tsp cinnamon
1 tsp nutmeg
1¼ cups rolled oats
¼ cup whole-wheat flour
2 Tbsp honey
2 Tbsp apple juice concentrate, thawed
2 Tbsp canola oil
2 Tbsp water

1. Preheat the oven to 350° F. Sprinkle the apples with lemon juice and add the spices. Place the apples in a casserole dish.
2. In a separate bowl, combine the oats and flour. Add the honey, apple juice concentrate, oil, and water. Work the mixture until it resembles crumbs and is moist. Sprinkle the topping over the apples. Bake for 30 minutes until topping is browned and apples are soft.

Starch Exchange 1
Fruit Exchange 2
Monounsat Fat Exchange 1
Calories 248
    Calories from Fat.................58
Total Fat....................................6 g
    Saturated Fat.......................1 g
Cholesterol ....0 mg
Sodium..................................4 mg
Total Carbohydrate ....47 g
    Dietary Fiber ....7 g
    Sugars..............................28 g
Protein ....4 g

Island Fruit Cup

24

How to Cook for People with Diabetes, p. 96

6 servings/serving size: ⅙ recipe

6 grapefruit sections
½ cup fresh or canned pineapple, sliced
½ cup papaya (or cantaloupe or other melon)
1 medium orange, peeled and sectioned
1 medium banana
½ cup diced mango (or cantaloupe or other melon)
2 tsp sugar substitute
1 drop red food coloring (optional)
¼ cup plain nonfat yogurt

1. Combine the fruits in a large bowl, then spoon into 6 individual serving dishes.
2. Blend the sugar substitute, food coloring, and yogurt. Top each serving with a dollop of yogurt. Serve well chilled.

Fruit Exchange	1
Calories	66
Calories from Fat	0
Total Fat	0 g
Saturated Fat	0 g
Cholesterol	0 mg
Sodium	8 mg
Total Carbohydrate	16 g
Dietary Fiber	2 g
Protein	1 g

How to Cook for People with Diabetes, p. 37

4 servings/serving size: ¼ recipe

½ cup orange juice
1 Tbsp vinegar
1 Tbsp fresh mint leaves
2 tsp sugar substitute
3 cups raw cabbage, shredded
4 Tbsp raisins
1 cup fresh orange sections, chopped

1. Place the orange juice, vinegar, mint leaves, and sugar substitute in a blender or food processor. Process the dressing for a few seconds, until the mint leaves are finely chopped.
2. Place the shredded cabbage in a large bowl. Pour the salad dressing over the cabbage and toss well to coat. Garnish with raisins and orange sections.

Fruit Exchange 1
Vegetable Exchange...................1
Calories....................................80
   Calories from Fat..................0
Total Fat...............................0 g
   Saturated Fat.....................0 g
Cholesterol ....0 mg
Sodium..............................11 mg
Total Carbohydrate ....20 g
   Dietary Fiber ....3 g
Protein ....2 g

Flavorful Seasons Cookbook, p. 205

6 servings/serving size: ½ cup

1 medium papaya, peeled and thinly sliced
2 medium mangoes, peeled and cut into 2-inch cubes
¼ cup fresh lime juice
2 tsp sugar

1. On a platter, place the papaya slices in a circular fan pattern. Pile the mango chunks in the center of the papayas.
2. Combine the lime juice and sugar and stir until the sugar is dissolved. Sprinkle the mixture over the papayas and mangoes and serve.

Fruit Exchange	1½
Calories	87
Calories from Fat	3
Total Fat	0 g
Saturated Fat	0 g
Cholesterol	0 mg
Sodium	3 mg
Total Carbohydrate	23 g
Dietary Fiber	3 g
Sugars	18 g
Protein	1 g

Brand-Name Diabetic Meals in Minutes, p. 35

4 servings/serving size: 1 cup + 2 Tbsp

8 oz frozen cheese-filled tortellini (about 2 cups)
½ cup refrigerated Marie's Zesty Fat Free Italian Vinaigrette
1 small cucumber, diced (about 1 cup)
1 medium tomato, diced (about 1 cup)
1 green onion, sliced (about 2 Tbsp)
Assorted salad greens (optional)

1. Cook tortellini according to package directions. Drain in colander. In medium bowl, toss hot tortellini with vinaigrette; cool 10 minutes.
2. Add cucumber, tomato, and onion; toss gently to coat. Serve at room temperature or cover and refrigerate until serving time. Serve on salad greens. If desired, garnish with plum tomato and fresh sage.

Starch Exchange	1½
Vegetable Exchange	1
Fat Exchange	½
Calories	168
Calories from Fat	30
Total Fat	3 g
Saturated Fat	1 g
Cholesterol	20 mg
Sodium	339 mg
Total Carbohydrate	29 g
Dietary Fiber	1 g
Sugars	5 g
Protein	6 g

Recipe provided courtesy of Campbell Soup Company.

Flavorful Seasons Cookbook, p. 63

6 servings/serving size: 1 small potato

6 small russet potatoes
2 Tbsp olive oil
¼ cup dry white wine
10 sprigs fresh rosemary
10 sprigs fresh thyme
Fresh ground pepper and salt to taste

1. Preheat the oven to 350° F. Cut each potato in half and place in a baking dish.
2. Cover the potatoes with oil, wine, herbs, pepper, and salt. Cover and bake for 1 hour.
3. Uncover and bake for 10 more minutes.

Starch Exchange 1
Monounsat Fat Exchange 1
Calories 114
   Calories from Fat................41
Total Fat..................................5 g
Saturated Fat ....1 g
Cholesterol ....0 mg
Sodium..................................28 mg
Total Carbohydrate ....17 g
   Dietary Fiber ....2 g
   Sugars..................................1 g
Protein ....2 g

Flavorful Seasons Cookbook, p. 198

6 servings/serving size: 1 cup

2 cups diced cooked chicken breast
½ cup celery, chopped
½ cup mango, chopped
¼ cup water chestnuts, sliced
2 cups pineapple, canned and drained or fresh, diced
1 cup mandarin oranges, in their own juice and drained
¼ cup low-fat mayonnaise
2 Tbsp low-fat sour cream
1 tsp coconut extract

1. Combine all ingredients and refrigerate for 1–2 hours before serving.

Fruit Exchange	1
Very Lean Meat Exchange	1
Fat Exchange	½
Calories	156
Calories from Fat	27
Total Fat	3 g
Saturated Fat	1 g
Cholesterol	42 mg
Sodium	143 mg
Total Carbohydrate	17 g
Dietary Fiber	2 g
Sugars	14 g
Protein	16 g

Appendix D

Resource List

Self-Care Titles

NEW! *Diabetes A to Z, 3rd Edition*
In clear, simple terms, you'll learn all about diabetes and blood sugar, complications, diet, exercise, heart disease, insulin, kidney disease, meal planning, pregnancy, sex, weight loss, and much more. Alphabetized for quick reference. Softcover. #CGFDAZ
Nonmember: $11.95/ADA Member: $9.95

NEW! *Type 2 Diabetes: Your Healthy Living Guide, 2nd Edition*
A thorough guide to staying healthy with type 2 diabetes—everything from choosing a health care team, eating, and exercising to self-monitoring, insulin, dealing with complications, and keeping mentally fit. You'll also find helpful tips on employment and health insurance. Softcover. #CTIIHG
Nonmember: $16.95/ADA Member: $14.95

NEW! *The Ten Keys to Helping Your Child Grow Up With Diabetes*
Here's help for parents who face the problems, feelings, and situations that can accompany managing diabetes. *Ten Keys* is a practical book for parents and care-givers of children with diabetes that addresses in detail the psychological, social, and emotional hurdles that often complicate the lives of youngsters with diabetes. Softcover. #CSMTK
Nonmember: $14.95/ADA Member: $13.95

NEW! *Women & Diabetes*
Designed for women, this book is filled with complete, thorough, and up-to-date discussions about a broad range of real-life topics such PMS, lactation, sex, pregnancy, child rearing, and menopause and the emotions that accompany them. Also includes dozens of checklists, charts, and exercises to help you create an individualized roadmap to living a healthy life with diabetes. Softcover. #CSMWD
Nonmember: $14.95/ADA Member: $13.95

NEW! *American Diabetes Association Complete Guide to Diabetes*
Every area of self-care is covered in this ultimate diabetes reference for your home.
You can solve problems with hundreds of hints, tips, and tricks that are proven to
work. It covers insulin use. Blood sugar control. Sex and pregnancy. Eating and
weight control. Insurance. Every aspect of your daily and professional life with dia-
betes. Paperback. #CSMCGDP
Nonmember: $19.95/ADA Member: $17.95
Hardcover. #CSMCGD
Nonmember: $29.95/ADA Member: $25.95

101 Tips for Staying Healthy with Diabetes
Get the inside track on the latest tips, techniques, and strategies for preventing and
treating diabetes complications. You'll learn everyday methods such as how to treat
and prevent skin infections, which cold and flu medicines to avoid, and how to eat
the foods you like healthfully. Softcover. #CSMFSH
Nonmember: $12.50/ADA Member: $10.50

How to Get Great Diabetes Care
This book tells you what kind of medical care you need for diabetes. It translates the
ADA Standards of Care so you know what you and your doctor should be doing.
Includes discussions of the goals of treatment, how to choose and effectively talk to
your doctor, and more. Softcover. #CSMHGGDC
Nonmember: $11.95/ADA Member: $9.95

Sweet Kids: How to Balance Diabetes Control & Good Nutrition with Family Peace
This new guide addresses behavioral and developmental issues of nutrition management in the families of children with diabetes. Each chapter begins with a story of a
child with diabetes to help introduce you to each topic. Softcover. #CSMSK
Nonmember: $14.95/ADA Member: $11.95

Reflections on Diabetes
A collection of stories written by people who have learned from the experience of
living with the disease. Selected from the *Reflections* column of *Diabetes Forecast* magazine. Softcover. #CSMROD
Nonmember: $9.95/ADA Member: $8.95

101 Tips for Improving Your Blood Sugar
101 Tips offers a practical, easy-to-follow roadmap to tight blood sugar control. One
question appears on each page, with the answers or "tips" below each question. Tips on
diet, exercise, travel, weight loss, insulin, illness, and more. Softcover. #CSMTBBGC
Nonmember: $12.50/ADA Member: $10.50

Managing Diabetes on a Budget
For less than $10 you can begin saving hundreds and hundreds on your diabetes
self-care. An inexpensive, sure-fire collection of tips and hints to save you money
on everything from medications and diet to exercise and health care. Softcover.
#CSMMDOAB
Nonmember: $7.95/ADA Member: $6.95

The Fitness Book: For People with Diabetes

You'll learn how to get your mind and body ready to exercise, exercise to lose weight, exercise safely, increase your competitive edge, much more. Illustrated. Softcover. #CSMFB
Nonmember: $18.95/ADA Member: $16.95

Raising a Child with Diabetes

Learn how to help your child adjust insulin to allow for foods that kids like to eat, have a busy schedule and still feel healthy and strong, negotiate the twists and turns of being "different," and much more. Softcover. #CSMRACWD
Nonmember: $14.95/ADA Member: $12.95

The Dinosaur Tamer

Enjoy 25 fictional stories that entertain, enlighten, and ease your child's frustrations about having diabetes. Each tale helps evaporate the fear of insulin shots, blood tests, going to diabetes camp, and more. Ages 8–12. Softcover. #CSMDTAOS
Nonmember: $9.95/ADA Member: $8.95

Diabetes & Pregnancy: What to Expect

You'll learn about the unborn baby's development, tests to expect, labor and delivery, birth control, much more. Softcover. #CPREDP
Nonmember: $9.95/ADA Member: $8.95

Gestational Diabetes: What to Expect

Discover what gestational diabetes is and how to care for yourself during your pregnancy. You'll learn about the unborn baby's development, tests to expect, labor and delivery, birth control, much more. Softcover. #CPREGD
Nonmember: $9.95/ADA Member: $8.95

Diabetes: A Positive Approach—Video

#CVIDPOS
Nonmember: $19.95/ADA Member: $17.95

1998 Buyer's Guide

#CMISBUY98
Nonmember: $4.95/ADA Member: $3.95

Cookbooks & Meal Planners

NEW! The Diabetes Carbohydrate and Fat Gram Guide

Calories are important, but knowing the fat and carbohydrate content of the foods you eat is the key to eating right. Registered dietitian Lea Ann Holzmeister shows you how to count carbohydrate and fat grams and exchanges, and why it's important. Charts list foods, serving sizes, and nutrient data for hundreds of products. Softcover. #CMPCFGG
Nonmember: $11.95/ADA Member: $9.95

NEW! Brand-Name Diabetic Meals

Save time cooking with these popular taste-tested recipes from the kitchens of Campbell Soup, Kraft Foods, Weetabix, Dean Foods, Eskimo Pie, and Equal. Features more than 200 recipes from appetizers to desserts that will help make your meals tastier and your life easier. Nutrient information included. Softcover. #CCBBNDM
Nonmember: $12.95/ADA Member: $10.95

NEW! *How to Cook for People with Diabetes*

Finally, a collection of reader favorites from the delicious, nutritious recipes featured every month in *Diabetes Forecast*. But you get more than pizza, chicken, unique holiday foods, vegetarian recipes and more, you also get nutrient analysis and exchanges for each recipe. Softcover. #CCBCFPD
Nonmember: $11.95/ADA Member: $9.95

NEW! *World-Class Diabetic Cooking*

Travel around the world at every meal with this collection of 200 exciting new low-fat, low-calorie recipes. Features recipes from Thailand, Italy, Greece, Spain, China, Japan, Africa, Mexico, Germany, and more. Appetizers, soups, salads, pastas, meats, breads, and desserts are highlighted. Softcover. #CCBWCC
Nonmember: $12.95/ADA Member: $10.95

NEW! *Southern-Style Diabetic Cooking*

This cookbook takes traditional Southern dishes and turns them into great-tasting recipes you'll come back to again and again. Features more than 100 recipes including appetizers, main dishes, and desserts; complete nutrient analysis with each recipe, and suggestions for modifying recipes to meet individual nutritional needs. Softcover. #CCBSSDC
Nonmember: $11.95/ADA Member: $9.95

NEW! *Magic Menus*

Now you can plan all your meals from more than 50 breakfasts, 50 lunches, 75 dinners, and 30 snacks. Like magic, this book figures calories and exchanges for you automatically. The day's calories will still equal 1,500 (or 1350 or 1800, depending on your needs). Thousands of combinations are possible. Softcover. #CCBMM
Nonmember: $14.95/ADA Member: $12.95

Flavorful Seasons Cookbook

Warm up your winter with recipes for Christmas, welcome spring with an Easter recipe, and cool off those hot summer days with more recipes for the Fourth of July. More than 400 unforgettable choices that combine great taste with all the good-for-you benefits of a well-balanced meal. Cornish Game Hens, Orange Sea Bass, Ginger Bread Pudding, many others. Softcover. #CCBFS
Nonmember: $16.95/ADA Member: $14.95

Diabetic Meals In 30 Minutes—Or Less!

Put an end to bland, time-consuming meals with more than 140 fast, flavorful recipes. Complete nutrition information accompanies every recipe. A number of "quick tips" will have you out of the kitchen and into the dining room even faster! Salsa Salad, Oven-Baked Parmesan Zucchini, Roasted Red Pepper Soup, Layered Vanilla Parfait, and more. Softcover. #CCBDM
Nonmember: $11.95/ADA Member: $9.95

Diabetes Meal Planning Made Easy

Learn quick and easy ways to eat more starches, fruits, vegetables, and milk; make changes in your eating habits to reach your goals; and understand how to use the Nutrition Facts on food labels. You'll also master the intricacies of each food group in the new Diabetes Food Pyramid. Softcover. #CCBMP
Nonmember: $14.95/ADA Member: $12.95

Month of Meals

When celebrations begin, go ahead—dig in! Includes a Special Occasion section that offers tips for brunches, holidays, and restaurants to give you delicious dining options anytime, anywhere. Menu choices include Chicken Cacciatore, Oven Fried Fish, Sloppy Joes, Crab Cakes, and many others. Spiral-bound. Softcover. #CMPMOM
Nonmember: $12.50/ADA Member: $10.50

Month of Meals 2

Automatic menu planning goes ethnic! Tips and meal suggestions for Mexican, Italian, and Chinese restaurants are featured. Quick-to-fix and ethnic recipes are also included. Beef Burritos, Chop Suey, Veal Piccata, Stuffed Peppers, and others. Spiral-bound. Softcover. #CMPMOM2
Nonmember: $12.50/ADA Member: $10.50

Month of Meals 3

Enjoy fast food without guilt! Make delicious choices at McDonald's, Wendy's, Taco Bell, and other fast food restaurants. Special sections offer valuable tips on reading ingredient labels, preparing meals for picnics, and meal planning when you're ill. Spiral-bound. Softcover. #CMPMOM3
Nonmember: $12.50/ADA Member: $10.50

Month of Meals 4

Meat and potatoes menu planning! Enjoy old-time family favorites like Meatloaf and Pot Roast, Crispy Fried Chicken, Beef Stroganoff, and many others. Hints for turning family-size meals into delicious left-overs will keep generous portions from going to waste. Meal plans for one or two people are also featured. Spiral-bound. Softcover. #CMPMOM4
Nonmember: $12.50/ADA Member: $10.50

Month of Meals 5

Meatless meals picked fresh from the garden. Choose from a garden of fresh vegetarian selections like Eggplant Italian, Stuffed Zucchini, Cucumbers with Dill Dressing, Vegetable Lasagna, and many others. Plus, you'll reap all the health benefits of a vegetarian diet. Softcover. #CMPMOM5
Nonmember: $12.50/ADA Member: $10.50

To order call 1-800-232-6733 and mention code CK997WLW

To join ADA call: 1-800-806-7801